Productive Living Strategies for People with AIDS

The *Occupational Therapy in Health Care* series

- *The Changing Roles of Occupational Therapists in the 1980s*
- *Occupational Therapy Assessment as the Keystone to Treatment Planning*
- *Occupational Therapy and the Patient With Pain*
- *Occupational Therapy Strategies and Adaptations for Independent Daily Living*
- *The Roles of Occupational Therapists in Continuity of Care*
- *Private Practice in Occupational Therapy*
- *Occupational Therapy and Adolescents With Disability*
- *Work-Related Programs in Occupational Therapy*
- *Occupational Therapy for the Energy Deficient Patient*
- *Occupational Therapy for People With Eating Dysfunctions*
- *Computer Applications in Occupational Therapy*
- *Sociocultural Implications in Treatment Planning in Occupational Therapy*
- *Sensory Integrative Approaches in Occupational Therapy*
- *Hand Rehabilitation in Occupational Therapy*
- *The Occupational Therapy Manager's Survival Handbook*
- *Certified Occupational Therapy Assistants: Opportunities and Challenges*
- *Occupational Therapy: Program Development for Health Promotion and Preventive Services*
- *Health Promotion and Preventive Programs: Models of Occupational Therapy Practice*
- *Developmental Disabilities: A Handbook for Occupational Therapists*
- *Occupational Science: The Foundation for New Models of Practice*
- *Occupational Therapy Approaches to Traumatic Brain Injury*
- *Productive Living Strategies for People with AIDS*

T𝑟 & A

Productive Living Strategies for People with AIDS

Jerry A. Johnson
Editor

Michael Pizzi
Guest Editor

The Haworth Press
New York • London

Productive Living Strategies for People with AIDS has also been published as *Occupational Therapy in Health Care*, Volume 7, Numbers 2/3/4 1990.

The Haworth Press, Inc. 10 Alice Street, Binghamton, NY 13904-1580
EUROSPAN/Haworth, 3 Henrietta Street, London WC2E 8LU England

Library of Congress Cataloging-in-Publication Data

Productive living strategies for people with AIDS / Jerry A. Johnson, editor : Michael Pizzi, guest editor.
    p. cm.
    Includes bibliographical references.
    ISBN 1-56024-024-5 (hard : acid free paper).
    1. AIDS (Disease) – Patients – Rehabilitation. 2. AIDS (Disease) – Patients – Services for.
I. Johnson, Jerry A. II. Pizzi, Michael.
RC607.A26P76   1990
362.1'969792 – dc20
                                             90-5274
                                                 CIP

Dedication

Each person with whom we come in contact makes a unique impact and contribution, sometimes without knowing it. I have been privileged to witness the courage, the dignity and the tenacity of so many men, women and children with HIV and their caregivers as they continue to impact upon and contribute to the lives of others. It is to those persons and to the memory of those who have journeyed before us that I lovingly dedicate this volume.

I also dedicate this to my dad and to the memory of my mom, who taught me service, compassion, strength, commitment and love. Their unending belief and support of my personhood and my work will always be the cornerstone for my faith and belief in the power of human beings. The cycle of contribution must continue.

Michael Pizzi

ABOUT THE EDITORS

Jerry A. Johnson, MBA, EdD, OTR, FAOTA, is President of Context, Inc., and Editor of *Occupational Therapy in Health Care*. She was Founder, Professor, and Director of the Occupational Therapy Department at Boston University (1963-1971), and more recently was Professor and Elias Michael Director of Occupational Therapy at Washington University in St. Louis. She served as President of the American Occupational Therapy Association for over five years and is a recipient of both The Eleanor Clarke Slagle Lectureship and the Award of Merit, AOTA's two highest awards. She serves as a national and international lecturer and consultant.

Michael Pizzi, MS, OTR/L, has been a leader in occupational therapy in the arena of AIDS care and management. Formerly of the National Institutes of Health where he developed a pediatric AIDS protocol and clinical programming for adults with AIDS, Mr. Pizzi currently maintains a private practice working mainly with hospice patients and those who are infected with HIV and AIDS. A frequent lecturer at universities and at state, national, and international conferences on the topic of AIDS and rehabilitation, he has co-developed with Mary Lou Galantino, MS, PT, a workshop titled "Transformation of AIDS: A Holistic Wellness Approach," a portion of which he was invited to present at the World Federation of Occupational Therapy Conference in Australia in 1990. Mr. Pizzi has written chapters for the first books on AIDS in physical therapy and in rehabilitation medicine. He is currently creating with Ms. Galantino manuals for clinicians, students, and educators in the allied health professions on the rehabilitation assessment and treatment of people with HIV and AIDS. Mr. Pizzi is also co-founder of Positive Images, Inc., an international educational consulting group and founder of The Retreat, a wellness program for those affected by HIV. He is a doctoral student in health education at the University of Maryland.

Productive Living Strategies for People with AIDS

CONTENTS

EDITORIAL

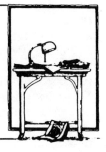

This work on AIDS represents the efforts of members of several disciplines (occupational therapists, physical therapists, social workers, nurses, and physicians, among others) who are involved in providing services to persons with HIV infections and with AIDS. It is interdisciplinary in nature and also covers the provision of many services to persons of all ages. It is well rounded in its scope and presents a holistic perspective in terms of both care and treatment of both patients and their families. Even professional readers may be struck by the consequences of AIDS, especially for those families in which both parents and their children have AIDS; rarely are parents confronted with having to plan for and face the consequences of a child's life-threatening illness or impending death while confronting and preparing for their own deaths or long-term illnesses.

The importance of acceptance and compassion is repeatedly emphasized by authors, as is the relevance of working with the "whole" person rather than with the person's disease. Professionals and others who work with individuals with AIDS face many challenges. These challenges include (1) the provision of support and guidance to persons who face long-term illness, disability and death and who seek to find peace and meaning in their own lives, (2) periodic acute care for opportunistic illnesses as well as rehabilitation services, (3) support and guidance for families, lovers, and friends, and (4) treatment directed at maintenance of function and participation in life. While the "treatment team" is important, each professional may also be called upon or required by virtue of circumstances to

1

fulfill any or all of these services. In many instances, an individual professional may also be experiencing personal grief, loss, and possibly helplessness because we have been prepared to physically heal or rehabilitate
our patients rather than to go through the process of dying with them.

While the focus of the book is directed toward treatment of persons with
HIV infections or AIDS, readers are gently reminded that as professionals
we must also take care of ourselves physically, emotionally, and spiritually so that we continue to have the creativity and resourcefulness to address many and varying needs, both our own and those of others. Sometimes this becomes a personal challenge for each of us. Meeting it also
will not only enrich our lives but those of others with whom we work,
play, and live.

Hopefully this work will contribute to each reader's life and work. It is
a reminder of how precious life is, and while affirming life, it reminds us
once again that the value of life is not found in its longevity but in its
meaning. Our greatest challenge is to provide the resources that empower
persons confronting devastating circumstances in their lives to find and to
create meaning that affirms their lives, sustains them, and makes possible
a satisfying and peaceful life and a gentle acceptance of death when its
time comes. By so doing, we, too, will learn to live and to die, knowing
that our lives made the world a better place for others.

Jerry A. Johnson

Preface

"Human adaptation falters when meaning cannot be derived from environmental interactions" (Reilly, 1974, p. 1). HIV infection and AIDS challenges human beings to adapt to the myriad of changes that it brings into one's life. These changes occur in the physical, psychosocial, environmental, cultural and spiritual domains of functioning. As these changes occur, meaningfulness of activity, of human relationships and of life itself is often questioned. Activities that were once carried out with ease during a typical day now require assistance. Independent functioning, that much valued commodity of human beings, becomes difficult to achieve on a daily basis.

This book is a commitment to independent and productive living for people with HIV infection and AIDS and their caregivers. Each article builds on the ones before it, acting as a team would when striving towards an Olympic gold medal. The intention of this book is to acknowledge the rehabilitation needs and examine the many possibilities rehabilitation intervention has for the person with HIV and AIDS.

Our journey begins with personal reflections of three persons affected by HIV disease. We learn HIV does not discriminate.

O'Connell explores the many medical aspects from the unique perspective of a physiatrist (a physician with special training in rehabilitation). He examines the medical dimensions of HIV and discusses the rehabilitation aspects of HIV, especially the need for occupational therapy (OT), physical therapy (PT) and speech pathology. I continue with the psychosocial aspects of HIV and explore the possibilities for occupational therapy programming with psychosocial dysfunction. Williams article continues that discussion and examines the value shifts experienced by people with HIV and AIDS. She discusses strategies for therapists to use in clinical psychosocial practice.

The article on culture calls for therapists to be sensitive to the cultural needs of people with HIV and AIDS. It examines the Black, Hispanic and Gay populations as subcultures of our society and concludes each section with clinical strategies. Spiritual values and spirituality are examined by an occupational therapist. The spiritual aspects of AIDS are discussed, however, unlike any other article on spiritual aspects and AIDS, Presti focuses on the spiritual aspects of occupation (life activity) and its powerful impact on the individual to whom it is applied. She also suggests that therapists look at treatment interventions used in psychiatry during the Moral Treatment era and their application to treatment used today.

Children with HIV are a growing population seen by rehabilitation specialists in clinics, school settings and in home care. Hinds-Harris and I, in the first collaborative OT and PT article on pediatric AIDS, examine the impact HIV infection has on growth and development. A taxonomy for pediatric AIDS is examined and strategies for OT/PT clinical intervention are discussed. The following article by Kaplan explores the myriad of psychosocial issues in pediatric AIDS. Hinds-Harris, Kaplan and I all believe in a systems perspective to care, that is, treating the family as the unit of care. This perspective is viewed in both articles.

Another growing population of people affected by HIV that needs attention is women. Wood and Aull do an exceptional job of exploring the facts about women and AIDS and examines the special needs of this group. Occupational therapy programming is explored, with an emphasis on concepts to assist women in maintaining their occupational roles in life and help them continue to be productive and active.

Men, women and children affected by HIV, at some point in the course of illness, may experience motor problems and pain. Galantino, a physical therapy pioneer in the area of AIDS clinical practice and research, describes some physical aspects of HIV, HIV pathology and several remediation strategies to restore physical function and reduce pain. She introduces concepts that are both traditional and nontraditional in scope.

The next three articles explore the many possibilities of program development. Schindler explores the extent of HIV and AIDS in the correctional setting, and describes clinical programming for people with HIV and for those at risk for HIV. Edson describes the St. Francis Center, a community support center in Washington, DC designed to meet the needs of people with life-threatening illness and the bereaved. Finally, Bonck and MacRae examine an adult day care program for people with AIDS and their caregivers. This model of care is an activity centered model primarily directed towards fulfilling the occupational and physical needs of people. Trends in health care today are pointing towards the need for alternative care for people with HIV and AIDS. It is my belief that day care will be regarded as a likely alternative for future management of the epidemic.

Throughout the course of HIV disease, people with HIV and their caregivers often experience multiple losses and changes which demand adaptation for survival. Okoneski describes bereavement uniquely related to gay human beings. She examines the multiple losses experienced due to

AIDS and acknowledges the unique aspects of being gay and bereaved. She presents a powerful case, in his own words, of a gay man and his struggle with his grief and his own survival.

The most rehabilitative and transformational aspect of our work is to respectfully treat each human being as an individual, with individual choices, values, skills, roles and interests. Dignified and respectful care can overcome the adversity and plight of so many and restore faith and hope in lives that may become meaningless because of HIV infection. Rehabilitation, combined with medical interventions, can make the difference between hope and hopelessness, power and powerlessness, and ability and disability. We must advocate for each other and for the dignity and respect for all humanity.

ACKNOWLEDGEMENTS

First and foremost I acknowledge Jerry Johnson, MBA, EdD, OTR/L, FAOTA and editor of *Occupational Therapy in Health Care*. When she first approached me with the idea for this volume, there was no hesitation in acknowledging the need for such a volume. What followed was an unbelievable amount of support and commitment to having this volume be an example of excellence for clinicians, educators, students, the lay public and people with HIV and their caregivers. I owe Jerry unending gratitude for her graciousness, kindness, commitment and generosity. I have the deepest appreciation for her as a therapist, a woman and a human being.

I also want to acknowledge the love and friendship of many colleagues, friends and particularly Mary Lou Galantino who saw me through this project. They were all understanding and reasonable when I was being unreasonable with myself and others out of my commitment to the excellence of this issue. I appreciate them all for the contribution they make to my growth and my life.

Michael Pizzi, MS, OTR/L

REFERENCE

Reilly, M. (1974). Play as exploratory learning. Beverly Hills, CA: Sage Publications.

Foreword

Productive Living Strategies . . . is a courageously positive title for this collection of papers by an interdisciplinary array of authors. Although HIV infection and AIDS, the subjects of their writing, are still considered terminal diseases commonly approached by preparation for dying, these authors prefer to view the illnesses of their patients more like chronic diseases that result in disabilities requiring multi-faceted rehabilitation interventions. Thus, from occupational therapists, physical therapists, social workers and nurses come practical, timely and appropriate strategies for holistic evaluation and treatment of the multiple physical and psychosocial problems faced by persons with HIV infection and AIDS. While representing different backgrounds, areas of expertise and treatment methods, the respective therapies present a uniform approach to their common mission in care and treatment: to alleviate their patients' psychosocial burdens of fear, guilt, isolation and loneliness, and to compensate for their losses of physical, cognitive and emotional function and independence.

All these therapist-writers also make a universal plea for attitudes of compassion, respect and dignity toward persons with AIDS regardless of the degree of variance with one's personal standards about sexuality, intravenous drug abuse and mortality. Repeatedly, the reader is asked to be sensitive to and accepting of alternative life styles; to avoid prejudice, bias and stereotyping of minority cultures; to support, not judge; and to foster positive approaches to improving the quality of what life remains. Such attitudes find close parallels in traditions of the Moral Treatment Era and in occupational therapy's concern for abilities rather than disabilities and shift of focus from illness to wellness. These views are re-emphasized in chapter after chapter, by first- and third-person accounts, through strikingly uniform descriptions of the broad-ranging effects of HIV infection and AIDS that restrict skills requisite to daily living and occupational roles; and of the many potential interventions appropriate for each weakness or loss that accompanies the inexorable progression of these diseases.

Health care professionals who are new to treatment of patients with AIDS-related conditions find frequent reassurances that their basic educational philosophy, principles and techniques of treatment are as applicable

7

for these patients as for others they have traditionally treated for developmental, neuromuscular, sensory, cognitive and emotional impairments. The core belief of occupational therapy in the effect of activity, or its absence, on health, plus the accent on function, independence and quality of life, are consistent characteristics of these writings. Inclusion of the patient, family, significant others and caregivers in treatment goals and planning are sound recommendations throughout the monograph.

A review of the Table of Contents reveals the comprehensive scope of subject matter, target populations, treatment settings and care provider perspectives addressed. Study questions at the end of most chapters test understanding of principal content. An appendix of national resources and additional readings provides a helpful supplement to the resources mentioned in, and the references which conclude, each chapter.

Author and Guest Editor Michael Pizzi is a leading proponent of occupational therapy for HIV and AIDS. In this compilation of papers, he has transformed a unidisciplinary concern into a multi- and inter-disciplinary focus on an increasingly serious health problem of the 1990s. To the extent that the disciplines involved assume the understanding attitudes and provide the practical interventions herein recommended, that problem can be significantly ameliorated for both those currently infected and the infinitely greater number of people at future risk for HIV infection and AIDS.

Wilma L. West, MA, OTR, FAOTA

Personal Perspectives

Mary Waterbury, MSW
Judith Williams, MSW, LCSW
Michael Pizzi, MS, OTR/L

SUMMARY. This article focuses on the personal stories, in their own words, of those affected by the human immunodeficiency virus (HIV). HIV does not discriminate, as is noted by the diversity of these personal perspectives. The authors hope that the reader will understand the many complex and varied issues that need to be addressed on an individual basis in assessment and treatment of people with HIV. There are no stereotypes of people with HIV. There are only human beings requiring dignified and respectful care and support.

PERSPECTIVE 1

Kevin

Kevin has hemophilia. In 1985, when he was 13 years old, his parents told him that the clotting factor which he regularly received to control bleeding problems had been contaminated with the AIDS virus and that he was now infected with HIV.

The majority of adult hemophiliacs are dealing with the same issue. The primary stressor in their lives is the ever present fear of developing AIDS. But like most adolescents, who feel that they are physically invulnerable—that "it can never happen to me"—Kevin rarely worries about becoming seriously ill. For Kevin, the most difficult aspect of being HIV+

Perspective 1: Mary Waterbury is affiliated with the Department of Hematology, Children's National Medical Center, Washington, DC.
Perspective 2: Judith Williams is affiliated with the Department of Social Work, National Institutes of Health, Clinical Center, Bethesda, MD.
Perspective 3: Michael Pizzi is in private practice and Health Care Consultant in chronic illness, hospice and AIDS in the metropolitan Washington, DC area.

9

is the sense of isolation which he experiences and which he sees as being almost impossible to resolve.

Kevin talks about his loneliness with the social worker at his hemophilia treatment center:

SW: "Are there people you can talk to? People who can give you support?"

K: "Not really. I can't talk to my parents. My mom acts like she can't stand to think about it, and she starts to get all upset if anyone brings it up. My dad just says 'Everything's going to be all right. They'll find a cure any day now' and goes back to watching TV."

SW: "What about friends?"

K: "Nope. Nobody knows. I mean, some of my friends know that I have hemophilia, and I'm sure they've heard about how some hemophiliacs have AIDS, but nobody has said anything to me."

SW: "Are there times when you'd like to bring it up yourself? When you'd like to tell someone?"

K: "Yeah, sometimes. There's this girl. She's the sister of a girl I used to go out with, and we're still good friends. If I told anyone, I'd probably tell her. But even if I wanted to tell someone, my parents would have a fit."

SW: "They're afraid of how people would react?"

K: "Yeah, they've heard all the horror stories. They think that somebody would come and burn our house down and run us out of town like those kids in Florida."

SW: "What do you think?"

K: "I don't know. We live in a pretty small town. People don't know much about AIDS, and most of them probably think you can get it from someone sneezing on you or something. So my parents are probably right."

SW: "So you feel you have to keep it to yourself?"

K: "Frankly, if it were up to me, I'd probably risk it. I mean, not tell a lot of people, but maybe a couple of friends."

SW: "What is it like, keeping it to yourself? How does it make you feel?"

K: "I don't know. It makes you feel like you're dirty or something. Like there's something so terrible about you that nobody can talk about it. I guess maybe I feel that way anyway, that having HIV means you're contaminated or something."

SW: "But talking to somebody about it, and being accepted by them might make you feel less like a leper?"

K: "Yeah, maybe."

Perhaps even more painful to Kevin than not being able to share his situation with his friends is his perception that he may never have a close relationship with a girl. It is difficult for him to talk about this. There are many stops and starts in this portion of the interview. Finally, he states:

K: "I mean, what am I supposed to do? Go up to a girl and say 'Hi, I've got HIV! Want to get into a DEEP RELATIONSHIP? At first, I didn't think it would matter that much. I figured that if I got close to someone, I'd just roll out the old condom and everything would be just fine. This was when I was younger, and I hadn't really started to try to get that close to anyone. I think I had this fantasy that when I met THE PERFECT WOMAN, she'd give me all this great sympathy and understanding."

SW: "And she wouldn't worry about getting infected?"

K: "I don't think I let myself even think about that."

SW: "And now?"

K: "Now I know that it just doesn't work out the way I thought it would. When I'm really with someone—with a REAL PERSON—I can't imagine her not freaking out! So what happens is, I get to know a girl just so well, and then I back off."

SW: "You just sort of fade into the woodwork?"

K: "Well, that's what happened at first. Like, I was at this party once, and I met this really cute girl, and we were having this great conversation, and I was pretty sure she liked me. And then I just went down into the basement and played pool with some guys for the rest of the night. Later, a friend of hers told me that she was really hurt."

SW: "So, on top of everything else, you felt guilty?"

K: "Yeah. So after awhile, I just gave up. I mean, I stopped talking to girls. I talk to them, but only, you know, kidding around. And if I see someone I think I might like to get to know, I don't even kid around with her, I just stay away."

SW: "Some guys would solve the problem by not telling the girl they were infected."

K: "God, I couldn't do that. I mean, what if something happened? What if she did get infected? Talk about guilt! And can you imagine keeping something like that from someone and always wondering what she'd do if she found out?"

SW: "She'd probably run away?"

K: "Yeah, and tell everyone she met on the way why she was running."

SW: "In taking the risk of telling a girl that you are HIV+, you're also risking her telling a lot of other people."

K: "Right. So now I just avoid the whole situation."

SW: "So you feel that you can't talk to your parents, you can't tell your friends, and you can't even begin to get close to a girl."
K: "That's about it."
SW: "It must make you feel terribly lonely."
Kevin shrugs, and says nothing, but his face is a study in pain.

PERSPECTIVE 2

Betsy

"My name is Betsy. I'm 47 years old, married, the mother of four, a third grade teacher in a local elementary school, and I have AIDS. I just don't fit the picture of an AIDS victim, and I think that is why the disease was not diagnosed for so long."

"In 1983, during the summer break, I had a hysterectomy. I had been bothered by fibroids and heavy bleeding which made my life miserable. My physician felt that I might as well have the operation, and since my husband and I were not planning on having any more children it seemed like a wise idea. I was enjoying my teaching and did not want to miss many days of teaching in order to have the operation so the summer seemed like an ideal time."

"The operation went well and I was recovering nicely but my hemoglobin was low, probably from blood loss the surgeon thought. He ordered a pint of blood to 'pick me up' and I must say I felt great after the transfusion. I went home after a week in the hospital and had no problems the rest of the summer. In fact, the next year was fine. I had the usual colds and one bad bout with flu, but otherwise no real problems."

"Soon after, I noticed that I seemed to feel tired a lot and I seemed to get every cold that was circulating among my students. My husband, John, thought that I was run down and he organized the kids to help out more with the household chores. My mother gave me an article about working women who try to be 'supermoms' as a not so subtle hint that I was trying to do too much."

"I must admit that I am a perfectionist and I set goals for myself and my children which are difficult to achieve. However, I have always been healthy and a hard worker. My kids are bright and I feel it is my job to motivate them and praise their achievements. All the children play sports and take music lessons. They have to be chauffered from one lesson or practice to another, and John and I take turns providing transportation. His younger brother is also involved in the business which was founded by their grandfather. The factory provides a modest income for us, but my paycheck helps to make our life comfortable. John has always been supportive of my teaching career and knows my commitment to my profession is important to me.''

"In 1985 I got real sick. I had a high fever and was hospitalized with pneumonia. The pneumonia lingered and after he had done every test and tried every antibiotic imaginable my doctor called in a consultant. At that time, reviewing my medical history, the consultant came upon the transfusion I had received in 1983. He suggested testing me for HIV. Well you now know that I was positive. The screening of blood for HIV was not started until 1985-86 and certainly very few physicians thought about HIV in 1983.''

"My pneumonia was pneumocystis carinii pneumonia (PCP), one of the opportunistic infections which occur when a person is immunosuppressed. My doctor told John and me that not only was I HIV positive, but that I had AIDS.''

"Well, this was the most devastating moment in our lives. I guess I was in shock for some time and I did not handle the news very well. I felt betrayed and angry and sad all at the same time. I could not understand how this disease which was so foreign to me and my community could have infected me. 'Why me?' I asked over and over. And what about John? Was he infected? We are normal sexually active people; I hoped and prayed that I had not infected the man I love.''

"I think my doctor was as distraught as I was when he learned of my disease. He may well have feared for his own safety. He had drawn many blood tests on me, done PAP smears and examined me gynecologically. He suggested that John be tested and also tested the children.''

"Now I know that it was probably unnecessary to test the kids, but at that time I didn't know very much about AIDS. I had thought it was a disease of homosexuals and Haitians and had no idea that it could infect normal people with unexotic lives. How could this happen to a straight, middle aged mother with four children to raise and prepare for the world?''

"I knew that I needed help, but I did not know where to turn. I did not seem to fit into any of the support groups that I read about in the literature my physician gave me. Then I contacted the AIDS hotline in a nearby city and they gave me a number to call for social services. There I was given your name and number as a psychotherapist helping women with AIDS. Our work together has helped me to live with dying. As you said, I am learning to live with dying. I can say it now, but you and I know how long it took me to accept that this is a terminal illness.''

"You helped John and me cope with this disease and all the stigma that our society heaps on those suffering from this disease. You educated us to not harbor anger and blame toward the homosexual community. We now attend a support group with Gay people with AIDS (PWA's), their lovers, family members, and two rehabilitated intravenous drug abusers and their families. John and I have grown in our tolerance since AIDS became a part of our lives.''

"We have passed the painful hurdle of telling our children and family. It was not easy, and we did not keep everyone together. My sister-in-law has never set foot in my house since she heard the news. She has shunned me, my husband and my children. It is hard for her husband, who works with John on a daily basis, and recently he has mentioned leaving the firm if John can buy out his share. The stigma is there, as is the need to blame someone and the fear of contagion. As you have told us, and we know it is true, we cannot spend the time we have left together worrying about those who reject us. We have too much to do to prepare our children and each other for the future.''

"I have had three more bouts with PCP since the first one when I was diagnosed. I have candidiasis and mouth sores and recently had a very painful case of shingles. The pain was unbelievable, but I have learned to live with pain. In fact, I will endure any pain and suffering to live. My youngest son is twelve years old now, and I would like to get him established in middle school before I die. I have left tapes for the children and told them of my love for them and my support for them in whatever they choose to do as adults. I am thankful for the time I have had to focus on parenting and getting close to my children, my husband and parents.''

"My mother and father are having a hard time, and they ask why this had to happen to me. 'My life is complete,' my father said. 'Why couldn't I take this disease from you so you could complete your life?' I don't have the answer to that and to many of the questions I am asked or that I ask myself. As you have told me, it does not help to ponder these questions except briefly. There are no answers, and there are other pressing responsibilities facing me at this time.''

"I am getting weaker, and although I deny it a lot I know that there is not much time left. I have worked out with John the plans for when I die. I have selected music for a simple memorial service for friends and family. I have written letters, mended all the fences that I feel strongly about, and can survey my life with some sense of accomplishment. I don't say that I have worked any wonders, but I have loved my husband and family, made a valiant attempt to rear my children and give them love and guidance of a good parent. I have been a supportive daughter and helped a lot of third graders look forward to learning and reading and the challenge of fourth grade."

"I am glad for psychotherapy and feel that it has enabled me to feel better about myself and to better accept this disease. There are many people living in pain with many illnesses, and many of them need help to go on with their lives. I am pleased that I didn't give up, that I lived my life to the fullest, and that even with a cloud of AIDS over my head, I was able to look up and see the sun peek through."

PERSPECTIVE 3

Mark's Mom

Dear Therapists:

Unfortunately, due to the hysteria that can arise from misinformation, I have elected to write you rather than talk to you in person. I have also elected to change my son's name in this letter. Having a family member with this disease puts us in a difficult position; however, we realize we have nothing to be ashamed of. Our wish now is to protect ALL of our children from discrimination.

Almost 2 years ago, our son was diagnosed as being HIV positive. Needless to say we were in shock and couldn't believe what the doctors were telling us. It took my husband and me at least a month before we could come to grips with this and tell our families. We have told all adults in both families although there are people that decide to tell no one. Our families knew that Mark was having problems, and we felt they deserved an answer as much as we did. Only a very few friends know of Mark's diagnosis. Some of these people have been very supportive while others are cool towards us. We accept these feelings and pray that someday everyone will understand that support and care help all of us to cope.

We've learned to deal with this illness one day at a time. It doesn't do any good to look at the past and ask "What if . . . ." Nothing can be changed now. As to looking to the future, I often think of my father's favorite saying. It is "We know not what tomorrow holds, but we know Who holds tomorrow." None of us knows what is in our future, but I do know that Mark has a better chance at having a future now that he is under treatment.

Mark, who is now 6 years old, was born prematurely after I had problems with the pregnancy. His lungs were not fully developed and he spent 10 days in neonatal intensive care. During this time he received blood twice. One of these transfusions carried the AIDS virus. At that time, replacement blood was given as a standard procedure once a certain percentage of the baby's blood was taken for tests. There was no need for permission to be given. Thinking back, most parents would have agreed to the transfusions if it meant keeping their baby alive.

Mark seemed slower to crawl, walk and talk than our other children. We were assured by numerous doctors that this was probably due to his prematurity. At two years of age, Mark was a fairly normal 'terrible two.' His speech was still very delayed, and what he said wasn't easy to understand. We were told this was because he had been intubated, had numerous ear infections or because his siblings did all the talking for him. (At the age of about fifteen months he had tubes put in his ears which put an end to the ear infections for a time).

At around the age of three, Mark spent about nine months in speech therapy. During this time, he was also hospitalized for pneumonia and reactions to drugs. The speech therapy seemed to help but there were still no answers as to why he was being so sick. By late 1986, Mark had a decline in the speech he had learned and a decline in his energy. When he was diagnosed a few months later, he didn't talk at all and would walk up the steps but not down them.

Shortly after being diagnosed, we found out about the program to treat children with AZT at a research hospital. When Mark was finally accepted, he had a very bad time. He would do nothing except lay on your stomach or shoulder. Feeding him became a problem as he didn't want to eat and you had to hold him on your lap while you fed him. It was about this time that we met Mike.

He and the physical therapist would help us with range of motion exercises to help Mark from becoming stiff. [Note: Occupational therapy treatment consisted of neurodevelopmental treatment and play activities to facilitate normal tone and reflex integration]. I believe this helped him in his eventually beginning to walk again. (No one is sure why Mark quit walking. It may have been the virus or a reaction to the drug.) When he began to walk again, Mark looked very much like the man in the television commercial who hadn't had his V-8 for the day. At this time, Mark would not cross midline with his arms and he had a problem with his wrists always being turned down. Mike worked with Mark and taught him the sign (in sign language) for love. This sign puts opposite hands on shoulders with arms crossing your chest. When Mark could accomplish this, Mike and I both had tears in our eyes knowing that he had improved and that he would finally be on his way to learning sign language.

When Mark was diagnosed, he was in a handicapped preschool setting sponsored by the school district. He was tutored at home for the remainder of the year and the entire following year. His teacher during this time was a real friend to me. She was one who saw improvement constantly and kept up our hope for the future. She was one of the few people in the school area at that time that didn't seem to be afraid to work with Mark.

Since beginning treatment (on AZT), Mark's progress has been astounding. CT scans show that not only has his brain stopped degenerating, but has started to regenerate! Every educational and developmental test that Mark has been given since starting treatment has better results than the last. Mark has been admitted into school and is learning sign language. That's hard on us, for now we must all go back to school to learn this foreign language!

The school district that we live in requires a meeting of all principal people involved in Mark's schooling every six months. As time goes by, these meetings are much less nerve wracking than the first ones were. I feel we have broken ground for the children who will surely follow in Mark's path. The school has been wonderful in keeping with the confidentiality that this matter requires. There are still problems, but they are diminishing.

Mark has learned that people understand the written word better than signing and will write notes to people. Recipients of his notes have been in church, restaurants and at school. Even Mickey Mouse and the Easter Bunny have been given special notes. His wrists are still stiff, but his signing is OK. Mike had made splints for Mark to wear at night. This seemed to help until he couldn't keep them on in his sleep. We work on exercising his wrists anytime and anywhere.

This letter is hard to write because it has brought back some hurt and sadness. On the other hand, it has reminded us of the progress that ALL of us have made. We realize that, without the help of so many people, our family would not be doing as well as it is today. We appreciate those who take an interest and treat our son as any other child. This is the most we can hope for our son and the other children who are infected.

Give them all a hug. They cannot hurt you.

Thank you.

A Mom

AIDS:
A Medical Rehabilitation Perspective

Paul G. O'Connell, MB, BCh

SUMMARY. This chapter gives a concise overview of the Acquired Immunodeficiency Syndrome (AIDS), with special emphasis on clinical aspects relevant to rehabilitation professionals. AIDS is a novel form of an acquired immune deficit now known to be caused by the recently recognized Human Immunodeficiency Virus (HIV). Symptoms result from the direct effects of the virus on the immune system and the nervous system, which appear to be the primary targets. Much of the morbidity and mortality, however, is caused by opportunistic infections which occur in patients unable to mobilize the appropriate immune defenses against them. Characteristic, but previously rare, neoplasms also occur due to a failure of immune regulation. Improved medical care, however, has changed AIDS from a rapidly fatal disease to one where survival may be prolonged.

The rehabilitation setting, the physical disability caused by AIDS, along with the psychosocial and economic impact of the disease on the patient have become increasingly important. Fatigue, decreased endurance, weight loss, edema, blindness and swallowing difficulties may all contribute to functional impairment. Neurological involvement is frequent and may cause dementia, hemiplegia, spastic paraparesis, painful neuropathies and proximal or distal muscle weakness. The clinical features and functional impact of these symptoms on the patient with AIDS is discussed, and the appropriate rehabilitation interventions outlined. Psychosocial and vocational issues are addressed as they pertain to the different clinical presentations.

Paul G. O'Connell is Senior Staff Physiatrist, Department of Rehabilitation Medicine, National Institutes of Health, Bethesda, MD and Clinical Assistant Professor, Department of Medicine, Georgetown University Medical Center, Washington, DC.

19

INTRODUCTION

When AIDS was first described in 1981 it was a rapidly fatal disease (Masur et al., 1981; Gottleib et al., 1981). With the knowledge and experience gained over the last decade, AIDS has now become for many patients a chronic disease with rapid fluctuations in their physical and functional status. As patients live longer, maintaining them as functioning individuals within society becomes important both for the individual and for society. Cost factors alone dictate this. Between one and one and a half million Americans are infected with HIV and are ultimately expected to develop AIDS (Heyward & Curran, 1988). The lifetime cost of treating a patient with AIDS is estimated to at least $60,000 and most estimates are much higher (Fineberg, 1988). Thus, keeping patients out of hospitals and functioning in society is in the interests of all.

Both the medical and rehabilitation communities have been slow to recognize that rehabilitation has a place in the care of these patients. The impetus for involvement has come from those rehabilitation professionals in acute care settings who found they were being asked to see and treat patients with AIDS (Galantino & Levy, 1988; Merritt et al., 1988; Pizzi, 1988; Pizzi, 1989). At least one institution now has a defined AIDS rehabilitation consult service (O'Dell et al., 1989).

AIDS poses a new challenge to rehabilitation professionals working in acute care settings. There is a real potential for rehabilitation to enhance the physical and emotional quality of life for patients with AIDS (Galantino & Spence, 1988). However, the goals and methods of intervention must be tailored to the needs of this particular population, which has neither the time nor the energy to devote to a traditional rehabilitation program.

In trying to establish a model of rehabilitation for AIDS patients an approach similar to that established for cancer rehabilitation is probably most appropriate. However, there are real differences compared to cancer rehabilitation. The AIDS population is quite different, comprising usually younger homosexual men, drug abusers, and children born to HIV-infected mothers, along with a dwindling number of individuals infected via blood products. These individuals have different needs, different strengths, and different levels of social support compared to the typical, more elderly cancer patient. In addition, the reaction of society to these people and to the diagnosis of AIDS is quite different.

The physical manifestations of AIDS, which are the primary focus of this article, are similar to cancer, multiple sclerosis, and other chronic progressive diseases in which rehabilitation intervention is now accepted as indicated. If rehabilitation is to be effective in this disease, however, those involved must have an understanding of AIDS and the expected behaviour of the particular manifestations of the illness present in any individual patient. Thus the intent of this article is to give the rehabilitation professional an overview of the clinical features of AIDS and enough information regarding the prognosis and expected behavior of patients with AIDS to effectively design appropriate rehabilitation interventions. Approaches to particular problems are outlined.

HISTORY

AIDS was first reported to the medical community in 1981. During that year the unusual occurrence in young homosexual men of Pneumocystis carinii pneumonia (PCP), was noted (Masur et al., 1981; Gottleib et al., 1981). PCP, which was extremely rare, had previously been seen only in severely immunocompromised individuals. Also that year, the frequent occurrence of Kaposi's Sarcoma, a rare tumor usually seen in elderly men of Mediterranean descent, was reported in the same population, sometimes in association with PCP (Masur et al., 1981). It rapidly became apparent that a new and probably transmissable form of severe immune deficiency was occurring. It was characterized by the presence of multiple opportunistic infections, Kaposi's Sarcoma (KS), and autoimmune phenomena and occurred in sexually active homosexual men (Heyward & Curran, 1988).

Within a year the same constellation of clinical findings had been recognized in intravenous drug abusers and then in hemophiliacs and other recipients of blood products. As the clinical picture expanded, a prodromal period of malaise and generalized lymphadenopathy of variable duration was noted. In addition, the development of similar symptoms in infants born to mothers who had AIDS or who were intravenous drug abusers was noted (Heyward & Curran, 1988). It became apparent that the main routes of acquisition of the syndrome were via sexual contact, infusion of blood products, or vertical transmisson from mother to infant.

In 1984 a novel retrovirus, variably called Human T-cell Lymphoma Leukemia Virus Type III or Lymphadenopathy Associated Virus, was described, and it was confirmed that this was the virus associated with AIDS (Gallo et al., 1984; Laurence et al., 1984). The name has now been changed to Human Immunodeficiency virus type 1 (HIV). Since then there has been a steady increase in our understanding of how this virus is transmitted, how it infects cells and how it causes disease (Redfield & Burke, 1988). In 1985, with the development of reliable antibody tests for

HIV, screening of the blood supply was introduced with a dramatic reduction in the number of new cases of infection with HIV from this source (Bove, 1987).

In 1986 the Food and Drug Administration approved use of the first specific anti-retroviral drug, zidovudine (AZT), which prolongs life in patients with AIDS. Multiple other potential agents are now being screened and tested for usefulness (Yarchoan et al., 1988). No curative agent is currently available. In 1989 AZT was approved for the treatment of patients with early signs of immune dysfunction to delay progression of symptoms to full-blown AIDS.

With the lack of a cure and the increasing recognition that a vaccine is technically difficult due to the high mutation rate of the virus (Fischinger, 1988), the current emphasis is on prevention of transmisson of HIV. For people already infected, the goal is to prolong useful quality of life by the use of antiretroviral therapy, by treatment of opportunistic infections and neoplasms and by a comprehensive multidisiplinary approach to supporting and maintaining the patient in as functional and independent a state as possible (Sande & Volberding, 1988; Abrams et al., 1986).

THE HUMAN IMMUNODEFICIENCY VIRUS

HIV is a retrovirus, a member of a recently described family of viruses whose genetic code is maintained as ribonucleic acid (RNA). Once inside the cell, however, the virus uses the enzyme reverse-transcriptase to make a deoxyribonucleic acid (DNA) copy of it's genetic material in a reverse of the usual process of transcription from DNA to RNA. The DNA copy is then inserted into the human genome where it is virtually indistinguishable from the host's own genetic material (Yarchoan et al., 1988). It then becomes dormant until it is triggered to produce viral RNA and proteins and to reproduce new viruses at the expense of the host's metabolic needs. These new viruses are then released to infect other cells. HIV must bind to the cell surface to enter and infect the cell.

The primary binding site of HIV is a viral protein, GP120, which binds avidly to the CD4 receptor found mainly on selected white blood cells. Because helper T-cells are the principal cells to express CD4 on their cell surface this makes them the primary target of HIV infection. Helper T-cells (also known as T-4 cells) are central to the immune response, influencing both cellular and antibody responses to infection and other immune challenges. Thus damage to them has a profound effect on immune competency. The fact that these T-4 cells, which are so vital to the immune system, are the primary target of HIV is what makes this virus so devastating (Redfield & Burke, 1988).

The T-4 cell is not the only target for infection. Cells of the monocyte-macrophage line are also susceptible to infection and may serve to disseminate infection to other organs such as the brain. The microglial cells of the brain, which are probably differentiated tissue macrophages, are also a target of HIV infection and may contribute directly to the encephalopathy encountered in these patients. This can occur even in the absence of gross immune dysfunction (Navia & Price, 1987). Bone marrow precursor cells may also be infected directly with HIV which may contribute to the troublesome anemias and cytopenias seen in many patients (Perkocha & Rogers, 1988).

PROGRESSION OF HIV INFECTION

AIDS is the final stage in the natural history of HIV infection. An acute febrile illness that resembles infectious mononeucleosis is recognized soon after infection in some patients (Redfield & Burke, 1988). This is usually followed by an asymptomatic phase of variable duration, although the development of AIDS within months of infection can occur. Usually tests for antibody are positive within several weeks of infection. It is now recognized that a number of patients may have negative antibody tests for a prolonged period despite evidence of infection in some circulating blood mononuclear cells. How likely these patients are to transmit infection is unclear.

Seropositive patients may develop generalized lymphadenopathy as their only clinical evidence of HIV infection during the asymptomatic period. After a period of months to years evidence of immune dysfunction occurs. This may be detected on laboratory evaluation (e.g., a falling CD4+ cell count) or seen clinically (e.g., cutaneous anergy) (Redfield & Burke, 1988). The development of chronic mucocutaneous disease, such as oral thrush, aphthous ulceration or herpetic ulcers, indicates a further progression of the disease and is a more ominous finding. Full blown AIDS is heralded by onset of a designated opportunistic infection or neoplasm. Some patients acquire neurological diseases such as HIV encephalopathy and dementia in the absence of obvious immune deficits (Navia & Price, 1987)

Two classification systems for HIV infection are available, but it is unclear if either has prognostic value greater than that afforded by measuring the absolute level of CD4+ white cells in the peripheral blood. A level less than 300-400/mcL is associated with a high risk of progression of disease. The Walter Reed classification system which has seven stages from WR0 to WR6, and the Center for Disease Control (CDC) system which has stages I-IV with subgroups, are shown in Tables 1 and 2.

On average it appears that it takes about seven to ten years for an adult to progress from initial infection to full-blown AIDS (Goedert & Blattner, 1987). There is tremendous variability, however, in individual rates of progression. In infants infected at or before birth, symptoms usually appear in the first two years of life. Once the HIV-infected individual has developed the clinical syndrome of AIDS, further life expectancy averages two to three years for adults and less for children (DeVita et al., 1988).

REHABILITATION APPROACH
TO SYMPTOM MANAGEMENT
IN AIDS AND HIV

The challenge in AIDS is to adapt rehabilitation techniques to a new disease. For rehabilitation professionals experienced in an inpatient rehabilitation setting where stable longterm disabilities are treated intensively, the change will be great. For those who are working in an outpatient or acute care setting, the change will be considerably less. AIDS has become a chronic disease in which rapid fluctuations in medical and functional status can be expected.

To plan interventions appropriately one must have a basic understanding of AIDS and the likely outcome of the current disease manifestations. Rehabilitation professionals who have experience in dealing with cancer, multiple sclerosis, arthritis and other chronic progressive diseases can draw on this experience to formulate approaches for the patient with AIDS.

Because AIDS may affect any system in the body, the rehabilitation team may, at different times, include physiatrists, physical and occupational therapists, speech pathologists, neuropsychologists, and social workers, among others. It is expected that Rehabilitation will be part of the support team rather than playing a primary care role.

Whether a patient is likely to improve greatly, get worse slowly, or pursue a rapid downhill course, will influence the approach. Interventions should be designed to achieve the greatest functional improvement for the time and energy expenditure put forth by the patient. Given the fact that these patients have limited endurance, take multiple drugs, and have multiple medical appointments and tests, their tolerance and cooperation for complicated exercise and therapy regimes is likely to be limited. Ideally,

Table 1.
WALTER REED CLASSIFICATION OF HIV INFECTION

WR 0	–	EXPOSURE
WR 1	–	ASYMPTOMATIC INFECTION
WR 2	–	PERSISTENT LYMPHADENOPATHY
WR 3	–	SUBCLINICAL IMMUNE DYSFUNCTION T-4 count < 400
WR 4	–	SUBCLINICAL IMMUNE DYSFUNCTION Partial cutaneous anergy
WR 5	–	MUCOCUTANEOUS SYMPTOMS
WR 6	–	OPPORTUNISTIC INFECTION

Table 2
CDC CLASSIFICATION SYSTEM FOR HIV INFECTION

Group	Description
I	ACUTE INFECTION
II	ASYMPTOMATIC INFECTION
III	PERSISTENT GENERALIZED LYMPHADENOPATHY
IV	OTHER DISEASE
Subgroup A	CONSTITUTIONAL DISEASE
Subgroup B	NEUROLOGICAL DISEASE
Subgroup C	OPPORTUNISTIC & SPECIFIED INFECTIONS
Subgroup D	ASSOCIATED NEOPLASMS
Subgroup E	OTHER CONDITIONS

rehabilitation services should be coordinated as closely as possible with, and be situated near, the sites of the patients' primary care. For some, home based therapy is likely to be the only option. Involvement of family members, lovers and others who play a significant part in the patient's life is often needed to accomplish the desired goals.

DISEASE MANIFESTATIONS OF HIV INFECTION

Every organ system can be affected directly or indirectly at some time by HIV. Symptoms may be caused by direct toxicity of the virus on an organ system. Much of the neurological disease is of this type. Malabsorbtion and diarrhea may also result from direct involvement of the gastrointestinal system.

Early on in HIV infection, autoimmune diseases usually associated with a hyperactive immmune system may occur. Guillain-Barre type acute polyneuropathy is an example of this and has been described as a first clinical manifestation of HIV infection (Cornblath et al., 1987). Immune mediated thrombocytopenia and myositis have also been described. Most of the burden of disease however, is due to opportunistic infections or neoplasms which occur in the setting of HIV-induced immune deficiency. A summary of the most frequent clinical presentations along with others where rehabilitation intervention is appropriate follows.

CONSTITUTIONAL SYMPTOMS

Malaise and fatigue may be seen even before patients develop an AIDS defining disease or infection. Fevers, nightsweats and weight loss are also common and may be either HIV-related or due to superimposed infections (Abrams et al., 1986).

Once patients are symptomatic, weight loss is common and is variably contributed to by anorexia, malabsorbtion and the effects of systemic disease. Profound weight loss is almost universal in the late stages of AIDS. Fatigue and inability to cope with continued employment or activities of daily living such as shopping will eventually occur. Even in the absence of significant neurological disease, if weight loss is severe, weakness may interfere with basic self care, rendering patients unsafe in their physical environments, limiting occupational roles and total functioning.

Rehabilitation intervention depends on the extent of the fatigue and weakness present. Early on in the disease, review of principles of energy conservation, prioritization of tasks and work simplification by an occupational therapist may keep patients functional longer. When adaptation is impossible, changing living environments to eliminate stairs and other physical challenges and to increase proximity to needed services and supports should be considered while patients are still up to the effort of moving. Gentle conditioning programs to maintain muscle strength should be encouraged. In latter stages, adaptive bedroom and bathroom equipment may be needed for safety, and gait aids may be needed for ambulation. Supervised living arrangements, coordination of community services and home visits by health professionals and personal attendants may also be indicated.

PULMONARY DISEASE

In adult patients, most pulmonary disease is due to infections which may be protozoal, fungal, bacterial or viral, and which are usually acute or subacute events (Sande & Volberding, 1988; Devita et al., 1988). HIV appears to have no important direct effects on the pulmonary system in adults. In children an indolent process called lymphoid interstitial pneumonitis (LIP) is frequently seen. The Epstein-Barr virus (EBV) has been implicated as the etiological agent in LIP, perhaps in association with HIV (Sande, 1988).

Pneumocystis carinii pneumonia (PCP) is the most important opportunistic pulmonary infection (Masur & Kovacs, 1988). Sixty percent of patients present with PCP as their AIDS-defining illness. Ultimately, eighty percent will have one or more episodes of PCP during the course of their illnesses (Masur & Kovacs, 1988). It is a major cause of morbidity and death in AIDS. Symptoms can range from cough and fever to fulminant respiratory failure. Typically, patients are breathless and distressed and have frothy sputum. Physical examination of the lungs may show little to clinically suggest pneumonia. Treatment is with trimethoprim-sulphamethoxazole (Bactrim/Septrim), or pentamadine, and response is better in early treatment. Chronic prophylaxis with oral or aerosolized medication is indicated to prevent recurrence.

The incidence of tuberculosis (TB) has risen dramatically in areas of high HIV prevalence, and in some TB clinics 50% of new patients are seropositive for HIV. Immune deficiency and possibly transmission via inhalation devices used for aerosolized pentamidine are suspected as contributing to the spread of the infection. The greatest incidence of TB is seen in susceptible populations such as drug addicts and Haitians. Similarly the fungal infections histoplasmosis and coccidiodosis are increased in patients in endemic areas. Viral pneumonias due to cytomegalovirus

(CMV) and varicella, and other viruses are also increased in incidence. Patients are also prone to the usual bacterial causes of pneumonia.

In the recovery phase of pneumonias the rehabilitation approach is similar to that outlined above for constitutional symptoms, with the addition that supervised programs of conditioning exercises may be needed to regain needed endurance and strength. As soon as patients are stable and capable of getting out of their hospital beds progressive mobilization under physical therapy supervision is indicated. Occupational therapists should review patients for changes in physical abilities and endurance that are likely to have an impact on their home or vocational situation.

MUCOCUTANEOUS DISEASE

One of the earliest and most frequent signs of clinical immune deficiency in HIV infection is mucocutaneous candidiasis (thrush). It is present in almost every patient who meets CDC criteria for AIDS (Sande & Volberding, 1988; DeVita et al., 1988). Other mucocutaneous lesions include painful perioral and perianal ulcers due to Herpes simplex, aphthous ulceration and non ulcerative lesions such as genital warts and molluscum contagiosum. Indolent lesions due to venereal diseases may be seen in perioral and perianal areas. Dental and oral hygene is often poor. Poor salivary flow and dry mouth resulting from involvement of the salivary glands is frequent and compounds the problem. Oral lesions may make chewing and swallowing difficult or painful and interfere with taste and enjoyment of food. Favoured hot or spicy foods may have to be avoided along with chewy or textured foods. It is often necessary for a dietitian to see patients to modify diet while maintaining palatability. As with esophageal lesions, oral lesions may occasionally preclude adequate nutrition and alternative methods such as supplements, tube feeding or parenteral nutrition have to be used to maintain caloric intake while dealing with the local problem.

For candidal and herpetic lesions specific therapy is available. Most patients with AIDS are on maintenance therapy with antifungal lozenges and receive acyclovir when indicated for herpetic lesions. Careful oral hygene, use of antiseptic rinses, and anesthetic gels or solutions are recommended.

Skin lesions such as dry, flaky skin and hair loss are almost universal late in the disease. Psoriasis, fungal and other skin rashes are common. Shingles due to reactivation of the Herpes zoster virus is common and painful and may be disseminated or multidermatomal. Hospitalization for high dose intravenous acyclovir is indicated in the latter case.

GASTROINTESTINAL DISEASE

Gastrointestinal disease that limits adequate nutritional intake is a major problem in late AIDS (Sande & Volberding, 1988; DeVita et al., 1988). Esophagitis caused mainly by candidal or herpetic infection can make swallowing extremly painful or impossible. Diarrhea and malabsorption are frequent and have multiple causes, most of which have at best unsatisfactory treatment. The protozoa Cryptosporidium and Isospora, mycobacterium avium-intercellulare (MAI), cytomegalovirus (CMV), AIDS enteropathy, Kaposi's sarcoma and intestinal lymphoma all may cause both symptoms. Colitis with bloody stool may be seen.

Functional impairment is usually related to weight loss and the weakness and decreased endurance that accompanies it. However, with chronic diarrhea, frequency and looseness of bowel motions and the need to be near a bathroom may, in themselves, be major functional problems limiting a patients vocational and avocational opportunities. Where specific treatment is lacking, symptomatic management with antidiarrheals and a major effort to maintain adequate calorie and protein intake are needed to prevent progressive weight loss. A combined effort of the occupational therapist and the dietitian to establish a manageable plan of meals, snacks and supplements that is appropriate for the individual patient may be helpful in avoiding more agressive nutritional supplementations, such as tube feeding and intravenous parenteral nutrition.

BLOOD DYSCRASIAS

Many patients with AIDS are anemic, have low platelet counts, and low white blood cell counts (WBC). They present with symptoms such as breathlessness, fatigue, decreased concentration, bruising and bleeding, and in the case of low WBC, increased infections (Perkocha & Rogers, 1988). Early in the disease auto-immune thrombocytopenia may present with bruising and bleeding. Later, bone marrow suppression may be due to HIV, other associated infections such as MAI, or treatment with AZT, or frequently a combination of all three.

Frequent blood transfusions may be needed to maintain an adequate hematocrit and control symptoms such as fatigue. Anemia and leukopenia are important side effects of AZT and are frequently the reason for failure to tolerate the drug. The absolute lymphocyte count and T-4 cell count are useful to follow progress of disease and response to treatments such as AZT. Low counts are associated with increased risk of opportunistic infections and poorer prognosis. Management of symptoms of fatigue and decreased endurance is as outlined previously.

KAPOSI'S SARCOMA AND OTHER MALIGNANCIES

Kaposi's sarcoma (KS) is a highly vascular tumor of uncertain etiology. It is seen especially in the homosexual AIDS population but can also be seen in all groups with the disease, although it is rare in children (Krigel & Friedman-Kein, 1988).

Skin lesions are present in 90% of patients with KS. These are raised purplish placques and nodules that are usually multiple and spreading, often coalescing into larger lesions. Initially they may be small and asymptomatic. If extensive, the skin lesions may be very obvious and readily recognized by those with experience of KS. For some patients this may pose major problems, especially if their work involves interaction with the public. Also, by identifying a person as having AIDS, cutaneous KS may contribute to his social isolation, either by causing him to be shunned or as a result of self-imposed isolation precipitated by embarrassment or fear. Indeed in our experience, the psychosocial impact of cutaneous KS may be the most disabling feature of having AIDS in some patients and may be the main thrust of rehabilitation intervention.

For patients reluctant to be exposed to the general public, modifications of work routines to allow work from a home setting using personal computers and telephones may be possible for a lucky few. For others, the therapist may devise home exercise programs and find alternative ways to increase outside activities in a protected environment (Pizzi, 1989). Counselling by an experienced therapist, psychologist or social worker can be helpful.

Physical problems may be caused by cutaneous KS lesions if they are in pressure areas such as the sole of the feet where abrasion, bleeding and superficial infection can greatly limit ambulation. However, it is the dissemination to visceral organs and lymph nodes that causes much of the associated morbidity. Obstruction of lymphatic drainage may cause progressive edema of the lower extremities and scrotum, causing difficulty fitting shoes and clothes, discomfort from stretching of tissues, and increased risk of superficial infections.

The weight of edematous extremities alone may be a burden for weakened patients which limits ambulation. Visceral KS occurs in most patients. KS lesions in the mouth, pharynx, and esophagus may make swallowing difficult or impossible. Involvement of the gastrointestinal tract may cause slow oozing of blood or interfere with absorbtion and nutrition. Pulmonary involvement is an ominous finding with poor long term survival. Survival is better if patients present with limited cutaneous KS and no opportunistic infections and is worse in the reversed situation (Krigel & Friedman-Kein, 1988).

Chemotherapy and use of biological agents such as Alpha-interferon may be of some use in disseminated disease. Radiation may be used to control locally troublesome lesions. Irradiation of the feet is very helpful for KS of the soles. Lesions in the oropharynx obstructing swallowing or respiration may also benefit from irradiation. In the short term, however, this may aggravate mucosal ulceration and dysphagia.

If skin lesions break down and become infected, whirlpool treatments may be needed to assist debridement and healing. Standards of disinfection for whirlpools after use must be established and followed meticulously. Lesions on soles of feet may require unweighting of feet via walker or crutches, the use of soft plastizote inserts to decrease friction and extra-depth or cast shoes. Control of edema via compression garments is needed when lymphatic obstruction or dependent edema occurs and may reduce the effort of moving heavy swollen limbs.

Other malignancies which occur with increased frequency in AIDS patients include high-grade lymphomas which present with advanced extralymphatic disease as well as with lymph gland swelling. The brain is frequently involved as the site of primary central nervous system (CNS) lymphoma (Navia & Price, 1986). The response to treatment is usually limited and prognosis is poor.

NEUROLOGICAL COMPLICATIONS OF AIDS

In this hospital the most frequent reason for rehabilitation consultation for AIDS patients is generalized weakness and deconditioning associated with systemic illness. The next most common reason relates to the neurological complications of the disease. HIV infection can affect any portion of the neurological system, including the brain, spinal cord, peripheral nerves and muscle (Gabuzda & Hirsch, 1987; Dalakas & Prezeshpour, 1988; McArthur, 1987; and Navia & Price, 1986). Table 3 shows selected neurological complications involving the brain, spinal cord and peripheral nerves which may benefit from rehabilitation involvement.

HIV ENCEPHALOPATHY

HIV encephalopathy (HE), also known as AIDS-related dementia, appears to be a primary infection of the neuroglial cells and monocyte-macrophages of the CNS. It may predate clinical immunodeficiency and is an AIDS-defining illness that is the presenting symptom in about 10% of patients (Navia et al., 1986). Prevalence of cognitive deficits suggestive of HE in patients with established AIDS is higher with estimates from 16% to 70% (McArthur, 1986; Navia & Price, 1987), with the higher

Table 3   COMMON NEUROLOGICAL COMPLICATIONS OF AIDS

BRAIN

HIV ENCEPHALOPATHY
CMV ENCEPHALITIS
PROGRESSIVE MULTIFOCAL
  LEUKOENCEPHALOPATHY
HERPES VIRUS ENCEPHALITIS
CNS TOXOPLASMOSIS
CNS TUBERCULOSIS
CNS LYMPHOMA

PERIPHERAL NERVES

DISTAL MOTOR/SENSORY NEUROPATHY
CMV POLYNEUROPATHY
VARICELLA/ZOSTER (SHINGLES)
DRUG RELATED (ddC, INH)
INFLAMMATORY DEMYELINATING
  NEUROPATHY
COMPRESSION NEUROPATHY
VASCULITIC NEUROPATHY

SPINAL CORD

VACUOLAR MYELOPATHY
VARICELLA/ZOSTER MYELOPATHY
CMV MYELOPATHY

MUSCLE

POLYMYOSITIS
TOXIC MYOPATHIES (AZT)
INFECTIOUS MYOPATHIES
  (Toxo, Coxsackie)
OTHERS

estimates usually indicating milder cases. Early features are memory loss, apathy, depression and difficulty with higher cognitive functions. Work difficulties may be seen where memory, concentration, judgement and skills such as language, visuo-spatial skills and math are impaired. Superficial testing of mental status is often normal in early HE, and detailed neuropsychological testing is needed to distinguish it from depression which it strongly resembles and which is also present in the same population (Navia et al., 1986; McArthur, 1987). In early disease, motor neurological deficits are uncommon, and patients are capable of independent self-care but may have trouble with instrumental activities of daily living (ADL) and financial matters.

In late HE severe dementia is seen. Memory loss is pronounced, cognitive deficits obvious, and speech may be disturbed. Neurological examination reveals spasticity, gait disturbances and hyperreflexia. Associated myelopathy is frequently seen. These patients are unable to function independently and need assistance or supervision in self-care. Bowel and bladder function may be compromised. Mean survival in early studies was three months or less at this stage; however, AZT may slow or even temporarily reverse the effects of HE in some patients (Schmitt et al., 1988). Mild symptoms of HE are common in late stages of AIDS, and indeed most patients dying of the disease show the characteristic pathological changes of encephalopathy (Grey et al., 1988).

Interventions in early HE include referral for neuropsychological evaluation of cognitive function to establish the types of deficits and suggest possible compensatory strategies. Recommendations may include use of memory aids, diaries and shifting from auditory to visual memory. Vocational counselling may be needed, and a lateral switch to a less demanding job may keep patients working longer. Due to problems with insurance, patients with AIDS rarely have the luxury of changing employers.

An occupational therapist (OTR) should review adaptive functioning at home and at work. This is the time to establish and review the patient's support systems and home environment with recognition that deterioration is likely. For mild and moderate dementia adaption of the home and establishment of structured routines by an occupational therapist can maintain patients functioning longer. The therapist may work to simplify tasks such as cooking and shopping, developing checklists and other safeguards to allow independent function to continue safely.

In late dementia, the patient's home support system is vital to keep him or her out of institutional care for as long as possible. Professional support from visiting nurses, social services or home health aids is needed frequently. Occupational and physical therapy (PT) home visits are often essential to evaluate safety in the bathroom and bedroom and for transfers and mobility. Based on this, adaptive equipment can be prescribed and caretakers instructed in supervision of safe transfers and ambulation using gait aids such as walkers.

Other diffuse CNS lesions are seen in HIV. Progressive Multifocal Leukoencephalopathy (PML) is a slow virus disease of the white matter of the brain that can cause dementia or focal CNS deficits. It has a more rapid course than HE. Encephalitis due to CMV, Varicella-zoster, Herpes simplex and other viruses may present also with diffuse CNS lesions. Allowing for adjustments imposed by the rate of progression of symptoms, an approach similar to HE is appropriate for all diffuse cerebral deficits.

CNS TOXOPLASMOSIS
AND OTHER FOCAL NEUROLOGICAL DEFICITS

Toxoplasma gondii is a parasite that causes focal cerebral abcesses which may be single or multiple in patients with AIDS (Navia & Price, 1986; DeVita et al., 1988). Lesions may be in the cortex, the sub-cortical white matter or cerebellum. Patients may present with headache, fever and confusion, but sudden onset of focal neurological findings are well recognized (e.g., rapid onset of hemiparesis). Findings will vary depending on the sites involved. Hemiparesis, hemisensory loss, dysphagia, ataxia, speech and cognitive disturbances are all recognized. CT-scans and magnetic resonance imaging show space occupying lesions in the brain with surrounding edema and compression of adjacent structures. Treatment with pyrimethamine and sulpha drugs, plus steroids if edema is present, may result in dramatic improvements.

As liquefaction necrosis of brain tissue may occur recovery is not always immediate or complete, and the clinical picture may be that of stroke in the young. Prognosis for these patients, if they can tolerate the drug therapy needed, is good in the short term, and they make very apppropriate candidates for accelerated rehabilitation programs, either on an in-patient or out-patient basis.

Early management while in the hospital is aimed at helping the medical staff define the neurological and functional deficits and avoid complications. As patients' conditions may be rapidly changing, it is important to be aware of potential difficulties with transfers, ambulation and swallowing.

Once these are recognized, nursing staff can be instructed in precautions for feeding, transferring and other activities. Once patients are stable, accelerated physical therapy, occupational therapy and speech and swallowing therapy can be commenced as appropriate. In our experience, deficits resolve fairly rapidly over the first few weeks following institution of treatment. After hospital discharge, outpatient therapy may be continued. In-patient rehabilitation rarely is indicated for more complicated deficits. Before discharge, gait aids and adaptive bathroom and safety equipment needs should be reviewed. For more involved cases or those with poor transportation, home PT and OT should be ordered.

CNS lymphoma usually has a somewhat slower onset than toxoplasmosis. However it can be difficult to distinguish either clinically or on imaging studies as scans may show exactly the same findings in either case. Patients may present with similar focal deficits, either acutely or subacutely. The prognosis for CNS lymphoma is much worse however. Radiation and steroids may provide temporary benefit, but following the initial improvement, a steady worsening may be expected in the patient's functional condition. The goal is to get the patient to maximum functional ability as rapidly as possible, using gait aids, adaptive equipment and compensatory strategies. Review of patients' support networks and home environment is advised, in anticipation of worsening functional status. PT, OT and other therapy modalities and social work should be involved as necessary, but clear, short term goals need to be defined.

Other focal neurological deficits in AIDS can be managed according to the basic principles outlined above with the approach tailored to the expected short term prognosis.

VISUAL LOSS IN AIDS

For any person, new-onset blindness is a major functional loss requiring great physical and emotional adaption. When it happens in the setting of a fatal disease, the impact threatens to overwhelm the patient's ability to cope, and much emotional and practical support is needed during this time.

Visual disturbances in AIDS are now increasingly recognized. CMV retinitis, which is cytomegalovirus infection of the eye, causes scotomata and blindness (Palestine et al., 1984). This is the most important cause of visual impairment although others are recognized. Treatment is difficult and unsatisfactory. DHPG, a neucleoside analogue not dissimilar to AZT, is the treatment of choice (DeVita et al., 1988). Patients may have to stop AZT to tolerate this drug. Thus, patients may have to make the difficult choice between a medication (AZT), their best hope for containment of their overall condition, and a medication (DHPG) which may help them retain sight. Unfortunately, progression of visual impairment despite treatment may occur.

Rehabilitation professionals can refer patients to organizations for the blind which teach techniques for blind rehabilitation. Patients are taught how to use a blind cane and instructed in appropriate modifications to their living environment to allow safe and independent performance of needed tasks. Talking books, large print books and magnifiers may be helpful. Referral to an OT familiar with ADL modifications for the blind may also be helpful. Learning Braille is not usually done beyond basic levels due to the time and effort involved. CMV retinitis occurs late in the disease process, and cognitive and memory deficits, sensory loss from neuropathy, or intercurrent illness are frequent impediments to successful rehabilitation of blindness. For parents and partners of the patient the impact can be equally devastating, and they may need emotional support as well as instruction in how to practically help their child or partner.

MYELOPATHY IN AIDS

Vacuolar myelopathy is due to primary involvement of the spinal cord by HIV infection and is seen in 11-22% of patients (McArthur, 1987; Navia & Price, 1986). It is strongly associated with HE. Vacuolar myelopathy presents with progressive paraparesis, posterior column sensory loss, and gait ataxia. Patients have spasticity and hyper-reflexia. Sphincter disturbances are frequent, beginning with urgency of micturition, and ultimately progressing to incontinence of bowel and bladder. Other causes of myelopathy include CMV, Varicella-zoster and Herpes viruses.

Rehabilitation management is similar to multiple sclerosis. Patients are provided with gait aids needed to maintain independent ambulation, including canes, forearm crutches and walkers. If foot drop is present, ankle-foot orthoses (AFOs) may be prescribed. Anticholinergics such as propantheline may be needed to inhibit urgency of micturition. Bedside commodes and bathroom equipment may help maintain safety and continence. A full ADL evaluation by OT with prescription of appropriate adaptive equipment is indicated. Solving problems associated with environmental difficulties, such as steps, is often needed.

PERIPHERAL NEUROPATHY

Peripheral neuropathy is an important source of dysfunction in the late stages of AIDS. The causes are multiple and are shown in Table 3 (McArthur, 1987). Neuropathy may present with problems due to dysesthetic pain, sensory loss or weakness. A distal sensory neuropathy is prominent in 30% of the patients (McArthur, 1987). It tends to be symmetrical and seen in advanced disease. Parasthesias and dysasthesias are common, along with reduced ankle reflexes and decreased distal sensation in a stocking and glove pattern. Ten percent of patients may present with painful soles and difficulty walking due to neuropathic pain and hypersensitivity. Frank muscle weakness is less frequent (McArthur, 1987), but atrophy of the intrinsic muscles of the hands and feet is not. When weakness is present it tends to be distal and presents as clumsiness and weakness of hands and as foot slap or foot drop. Proprioceptive loss may also impair balance. Depending on which is more prominent, the patient may have a steppage or wide based ataxic gait.

The drug dideoxyCytidine (ddC) which is currently experimental for treatment of AIDS, has been reported to cause an intensely painful dysesthetic neuropathy with severe hypersensitivity (Yarchoan et al., 1988). Rapidly progressive, severe neuropathy has been associated with CMV infection. This causes ascending paralysis of the limbs, progressing to respiratory paralysis and death (Eidelberg et al., 1986). Compression neuropathies such as peroneal palsy are possible in the acutely ill and bedbound but should be preventable.

Neuropathic pain tends to be a greater problem than weakness. Amitriptyline, carbamazapine, and phenytoin, all used in the management of other forms of neuropathic pain, have been tried in this situation with some improvement in symptoms (McArthur, 1987). Regarding physical modalities cold packs and vibration have been found to be most helpful. Transcutaneous Nerve Stimulation (TENS) and moist heat have not been too successful, especially for ddC neuropathy. For patients with hypersensitivity of soles, soft-soled shoes with good cushioning are recommended. We have made soft total contact orthoses for severe symptoms. Rehabilitation management of symptomatic motor weakness involves the use of gait aids and bracing of the lower extremities. Often, off-the-shelf AFOs are sufficient to control symptoms of foot drop. A cane or a walker may be needed for balance. Difficulties with fine hand function are due to either sensory loss or weakness. Appropriate adaptive equipment should be provided after evaluation by OT. For patients with stable weakness, a submaximal exercise program may be prescribed.

INFLAMMATORY DEMYELINATING NEUROPATHY

A syndrome of progressive motor weakness indistinguishable from idiopathic Guillain-Barre syndrome (GBS) has been described early in the course of HIV infection (Cornblath et al., 1987; McArthur, 1987). The pathology is demyelination of peripheral nerves, and it appears that the behavior of the condition is similar to idiopathic GBS. Most patients do not have overt signs of immune compromise at time of presentation. Rapid progression to AIDS does not appear to occur in most cases. Prognosis appears to be similar to idiopathic GBS, and a good recovery may be expected in many patients. General medical management and rehabilitation interventions should be similarly based on the clinical picture without regard to the HIV status of the patient. This is one situation where inpatient management on a rehabilitation unit may be appropriate.

Chronic and remitting/relapsing forms of inflammatory demyelinating peripheral neuropathy are also described in HIV infected patients (Cornblath et al., 1987; McArthur, 1987). These patients should also be treated based on their clinical picture and functional deficits.

MYOPATHY

Muscle weakness due to intrinsic muscle disease is a feature of both late and early stages of HIV infection (Dalakas & Pezeshpour, 1988; Gorad et al., 1988). Early on in the disease, an autoimmune polymyositis occurs which is steroid responsive. Like GBS, it does not reflect likelihood of progression to AIDS.

Patients present with proximal muscle weakness and raised muscle enzymes. Improvement is expected eventually, due to treatment or natural history. Late myopathy may be due to infection (coxsackie virus, HTLV = 1, and toxoplasmosis), toxic causes (ethanol, AZT), or autoimmune causes. Symptoms of proximal muscle weakness include difficulty in climbing stairs, getting up from a low chair or squat, or holding arms above head.

Patients may need raised toilet seats, bathtub benches and other adaptive equipment or gait aids to deal with problems. The role of exercise is undetermined. Vocational and avocational roles of patients with muscle weakness may be disrupted. Patients who perform manual labor or physically demanding jobs will be unable to perform their work and may need help in finding alternatives. Others will benefit from being taught principles of energy conservation and how to approach problem solving for their disability.

ARTHRITIS

The first descriptions of arthritis in AIDS were of a destructive lower extremity arthritis similar to Reiter's syndrome (Winchester et al., 1987). Reiter's syndrome is an asymmetrical arthritis affecting the spine and limb joints. "Sausage digits" and heel pain are typical features. In AIDS patients this arthritis appears to be particularly destructive and difficult to treat. An arthritis associated with psoriasis has also been reported (Espinoza et al., 1988). It is unclear if it is the typical psoriatic arthritis seen in individuals without AIDS. An acute arthritis that is severe but self limited has been described in patients with AIDS in whom no other etiology for symptoms was found (Rynes et al., 1988). Septic arthritis has also been reported.

Thus, arthritis in AIDS may be chronic or transient and of variable severity and mainly affects the lower extremities. Treatment includes physical modalities such as heat for pain relief, heel cups or shoe modifications for foot pain, splinting or unweighting of painful joints, and the use of nonsteroidal anti-inflammatory drugs such as ibuprofen. Patients may need to be taught the principles of joint protection and energy conservation.

CONCLUSION

This article has summarized the many clinical manifestations of AIDS, emphasizing those aspects that cause physical disability and have potential for useful intervention by rehabilitation professionals. Generalized debility and fatigue and the various neurological conditions that are associated with HIV infection constitute the two main areas where intervention is likely to be helpful.

Understanding of the clinical manifestations present in the patient being evaluated is important to setting realistic goals. While there is no cure for AIDS, improvement in treatment and survival times have caused it to behave more and more like a chronic disease which produces significant disability. Rehabilitation professionals working in acute care and home care settings can expect to see these patients as their numbers increase. Potential areas of intervention have been outlined.

STUDY QUESTIONS

1. *Name five primary medical manifestations of HIV disease. Name five rehabilitation needs of persons with those medical manifestations.*
2. *Develop a rehabilitation treatment plan for a person with: (a) Kaposi's sarcoma; (b) pneumocystis carinii pneumonia; and (c) upper and lower extremity neuropathy. Include physical and psychosocial types of treatments.*
3. *List ten strategies/modalities used by occupational and physical*

therapists that support people with HIV and AIDS in improving function.

4. *Describe the known routes of transmission of HIV infection, and list the primary social groups at risk of acquiring infection.*

5. *Describe the continuum of HIV disease from initial infection to development of AIDS. Develop rehabilitation strategies to follow this continuum.*

REFERENCES

Abrams, D.I., Dilley, J.W., Maxey, L.M., & Volberding, P.A., (1986). Routine care and psychosocial support of the patient with the acquired immunodeficiency syndrome. *Medical Clinics of North America, 70*(3), 707-720.

Bove, J.R., (1987). Transfusion-associated hepatitis and AIDS: What is the risk? *New England Journal of Medicine, 317,* 242-243.

Cornblath, D.R., McArthur, J.C., Kennedy, P.G., Witte, A.S., & Griffin, J.W., (1987). Inflammatory demyelinating peripheral neuropathy associated with human T-cell lymphotrophic virus type III infection. *Annals of Neurology, 21,* 32-40.

Dalakas, M.C., & Pezeshpour, G.H., (1988). Neuromuscular diseases associated with human immunodeficiency virus infection. *Annals of Neurology, 23*(Suppl), S38-48.

DeVita, V.T., Hellman, S., & Rosenberg, S.A., (Eds.)., (1988). *AIDS: Etiology, diagnosis, treatment, and prevention* (2nd Ed.). Philadelphia, JB Lippincott.

Eidelberg, D., Sotrel, A., Vogel, H., Walker, P., Kleefield, J., & Crumpacker, C.S., (1986). Progressive polyradiculopathy associated with the acquired immune deficiency syndrome. *Neurology, 36,* 912-916.

Espinoza, L.R., Berman, F.B., Cahalin, R.N. & Germain, B.F., (1988). Psoriatic arthritis and acquired immunodeficiency syndrome. *Arthritis and Rheumatism, 31,* 1034-1039.

Fineberg, H.V., (1988). The social dimensions of AIDS. *Scientific American, 259,* (Oct), 128-134.

Fischinger, P.J., (1988). Strategies for the development of vaccines to prevent AIDS. In V.T. DeVita, S. Hellman, & S.A. Rosenberg, (Eds.). *AIDS: Etiology, diagnosis, treatment, and prevention* (2nd Ed). (pp. 87-104). Philadelphia, JB Lippincott.

Gabuzda, D.H., & Hirsch, M.S., (1987). Neurological manifestations of infection with human immunodeficiency virus: Clinical features and pathogenesis. *Annals of Internal Medicine, 107,* 383-391.

Galantino, M.L., & Levy, J.K., (1988). HIV infection: Neurological implications for rehabilitation. *Clinical Management, 8*(1), 6-13.

Galantino, M.L., & Spence, D.W., (1988). Physical medicine management of HIV patients. In A. Lewis (Ed.), *Nursing care of the person with AIDS/ARC* (pp. 181-189). Rockville MD: Aspen Publishers.

Gallo, R.C., Salahuddin, S.Z., Popovic, M., Shearer, G.M., Kaplan, M., Haynes, B.F., Palker, T.J., Redfield, R., Oleske, J., Safai, B., White, G., Foster, P., & Markham, P.D., (1984). Frequent detection and isolation of cytopathic retroviruses (HTLV-III) from patients with AIDS and at risk for AIDS. *Science, 224*, 500-502.

Goedert, J.J., & Blattner, W.A., (1988). The epidemiology and natural history of human immunodeficiency virus. In V.T. DeVita, S. Hellman, & S.A. Rosenberg, (Eds.). *AIDS: Etiology, diagnosis, treatment, and prevention* (2nd Ed). (pp. 33-60) Philadelphia, JB Lippincott.

Gorad, D.A., Henry, K., & Guiloff, R.J., (1988). Necrotising myopathy and Zivudine (letter). *Lancet i.*, 1050.

Gottleib, M.S., Schroff, R., Schanker, H.M., Weisman, J.D., Fan, P.T., Wolf, R.A., & Saxon, A., (1981). Pneumocystis carinii pneumonia and mucosal candidiasis in previously healthy homosexual men: Evidence of a new acquired immunodeficiency. *New England Journal of Medicine, 305*, 1425-1430.

Grey, F., Gherardi, R., & Scaravilli, F., (1988). The neuropathology of the acquired immune deficiency syndrome (AIDS): A review. *Brain 111*, 245-266.

Heyward, W.L., & Curran, J.W., (1988). The epidemiology of AIDS in the U.S. *Scientific American, 259*(Oct), 72-81.

Krigel, R.L., & Friedman-Kein, A.E., (1988). Kaposi's sarcoma in AIDS: Diagnosis and treatment (pp 245-262). In V.T. DeVita, S. Hellman, & S.A. Rosenberg, (Eds.). *AIDS: Etiology, diagnosis, treatment, and prevention* (2nd Ed). Philadelphia, JB Lippincott.

Laurence J., Brun-Vezinet, F., Schutzer, S.E., Rouzioux, C., Klatzmann, D., Barre-Sinoussi, F., Chermann, J-C. & Montagnier, L., (1984). Lymphadenopathy-associated Viral antibody in AIDS. *New England Journal of Medicine, 311*, 1269-1272.

McArthur, J.C., (1987). Neurological complications of AIDS. *Medicine (Baltimore), 66*(6), 407-437.

Masur, H., Michelis, M.A., Greene, J.B., Onorato, I., Vande Stouwe, R.A., Holzman, R.S., Wormser, G., Brettman, L., Lange, M., Murray, H.W., & Cunningham-Rundle, S., (1981). An outbreak of community acquired pneumocystis carinii pneumonia: Initial manifestations of cellular immune dysfunction. *New England Journal of Medicine, 305*, 1431-1438.

Masur, H., & Kovacs, J.A., (1988). Treatment and prophylaxis of Pneumocystis carinii pneumonia. *Clinics in Infectious Diseases North America, 2*(2), 419-428.

Merritt, L., Smith, C., & Hirsh, D., (1988). Inpatient rehabilitation of acquired immunodeficiency syndrome (Abstract). *Archives of Physical Medicine and Rehabilitation, 69*, 716.

Navia, B.A., Jordan, B.D., & Price, R.W., (1986). The AIDS dementia complex: 1. Clinical features. *Annals of Neurology, 19*, 517-524.

Navia, B.A., & Price, R.W., (1986). Central and peripheral nervous system complications of AIDS. *Clinics in Immunology and Allergy, 6*(3), 543-558.

Navia, B.A., & Price, R.W., (1987). The acquired immune deficiency syndrome dementia complex as the presenting or sole manifestation of human immuno-deficieny virus infection. *Archives of Neurology*, *44*, 65-69.

O'Dell, M., Bohi, E., Schwartz, M.L., Wu, C.M., & Bonner, F.J., (1989). Disability in patients hospitalized with AIDS, (abstract). *Archives of Physical Medicine and Rehabilitation*, *70*(11), A5.

Palestine, A.G., Rodrigues, M.M., Macher, A.M., Chan, C.C., Lane, H.C., Fauci, A.S., Masur, H., Longo, D., Reichert, C.M., Steis, R., Rook, A.H., & Nussenblatt, R.B., (1984). Opthalmic involvement in the acquired immuno-deficiency syndrome. *Ophthalmology*, *91*(9), 1092-1099.

Perkocha, L.A., & Rodgers, G.M., (1988). Hematological aspects of human im-munodeficiency virus infection: Laboratory and clinical considerations. *American Journal of Hematology*, *29*, 94-105.

Pizzi, M., (1988). The challenge of treating AIDS patients includes helping them lead functional lives. *OT Week*, *31*(August 18), 6-7.

Pizzi, M., (1989). Occupational therapy: Creating possibilities for adults with HIV infection, ARC and AIDS. *AIDS Patient Care*, February, 18-23.

Redfield, R.R. & Burke, D.S., (1988). HIV infection: The clinical picture. *Scientific American*, *259*(Oct), 90-98.

Rynes, R.I., Goldenberg, D.L., DiGiacomo, R., Olson, R., Hussain, M., & Veazy, J., (1988). Acquired Immune Deficiency Syndrome-associated arthritis. *American Journal of Medicine*, *84*, 810-816.

Sande, M.A., & Volberding, P.A., (Eds.)., (1988). Medical management of AIDS. *Infectious Disease Clinics of North America*, *2*(2).

Schmitt, F.A., Bigley, J.W., McKinnis, R., Logue, P.E., Evans, R.W., & Drucker, J.L., (1988). Neuropsychological outcome of Zidovudine (AZT) treatment of patients with AIDS and AIDS-related complex. *New England Journal of Medicine*, *319*, 1573-1578.

Winchester, R., Bernstein, D.H., Fischer, H.D., Enlow, R., & Solomon, G., (1987). The co-occurrence of Reiter's syndrome and acquired immunodefi-ciency. *Annals of Internal Medicine*, *106*, 19-26.

Yarchoan, R., Mitsuya, H., & Broder, S., (1988). AIDS therapies. *Scientific American*, *259* (Oct), 100-119.

The Transformation of HIV Infection and AIDS in Occupational Therapy: Beginning the Conversation

Michael Pizzi, MS, OTR/L

SUMMARY. HIV infection and AIDS can be transformed through an attitude change and a change in thinking about levels of productivity and function of people diagnosed with HIV. This change in thinking demands that people with HIV/AIDS are viewed as vital, functional, productive and contributing members of society and the world. This article focuses on transforming HIV/AIDS through an examination of personal and professional transformation. It is through personal and professional transformation that the transformation of HIV/AIDS will occur. New ways of thinking about HIV/AIDS are explored. Present and future possibilities for therapeutic interventions are discussed. Transformation of HIV/AIDS will occur through empowerment of each other as human beings.

"A choice confronts us. Shall we, as we feel our foundations shaking, withdraw in panic? Frightened by the loss of our familiar mooring places, shall we become paralyzed and cover our inaction and apathy? If we do those things, we will have surrendered our chance to participate in the forming of the future. We will have forfeited the distinctive characteristic of human beings—namely, to influence our evolution through our own awareness." (May, 1975, p. 488)

Michael Pizzi is in private practice and is Health Care Consultant in chronic illness, hospice and AIDS. Correspondence may be addressed to the author at 8201 16th Street 1123, Silver Spring, MD 20910.

This article is reprinted from the American Journal of Occupational Therapy, March, 44(3), 1990, with permission from the American Occupational Therapy Association.

45

In her book The Aquarian Conspiracy, Ferguson (1980) stated, "anything that disrupts the old order of our lives has the potential for triggering a transformation, a movement toward greater maturity, openness, strength" (p. 73). HIV has forever altered the ways in which human beings think and act on life and living. Through an examination of HIV as an opportunity and possibility for personal and professional transformation, we can "influence our evolution through our own awareness."

HIV has had a profound effect on the ways in which communities, societies and the world cope with life's unknowns. HIV has provided us with a choice: As occupational therapists, we must choose either to remain, threatened, fearful and disempowered by the disease and its medical and social sequelae or to take action; to strengthen our personal and professional character, values and integrity; and to become role models in health care. The choice we make today will influence who we become tomorrow.

The conversation I am beginning is one grounded in several of my own beliefs. I believe that: (1) human beings have the power and ability to change and transform anything into possibility; (2) engagement in occupation is transformational; (3) occupational therapists influence the state of health of the people they serve through their own self awareness and their knowledge of the art and science of occupation; (4) occupational therapists have a responsibility and opportunity to transform the ways in which health care is provided; (5) human beings are deserving of dignified and respectful care provided in accordance with their individual choices and values; (6) open and honest communication amongst ourselves and our patients is essential.

PERSONAL TRANSFORMATION

In the HIV pandemic, fear often prevails, and it disempowers persons with HIV, their caregivers and the people who serve them. Personal fear requires transformation. Once this begins, societal and global fear can be transformed.

I believe that fear is a response to something uncommunicated and often unacknowledged, something perceived as threatening and confrontational, and something that is unfamiliar and that demands adaptation; all of these characteristics seize a person's control. HIV confronts us because it forces us to examine our personal values concerning homosexuality and bisexuality, intravenous drug use and our own mortality. The fear of contagion is linked to the fear of one's own mortality. As Frank (1958) said, "Man is always faced with the threat of obliteration, and this is probably the root of anxiety all humans feel . . . Man must construct a meaningful world out of his environment" (p. 215). We must examine these personal fears and values to transform our thinking about HIV.

HIV may make some persons uncomfortable because it challenges their vision of the "ideal self," "the person I would like to be or feel I ought to be" (Frank, 1958, p. 218). If we maintain a vision of who we ought to be, then we limit our ability to grow, to learn and to discover. Too often, we feel others ought to be a certain way. If we believe that certain types of people or behaviors are bad and wrong, it will affect our interaction with them. An acknowledgement of who the patient is rather than of who the patient ought to be can be powerfully transformative.

In patient-therapist interactions, we bring who we are, including our values, beliefs and interests, into the interaction. Our expectations, judgments or values and attitudes about homosexuality and bisexuality, intravenous drug use, and racial minorities affect our interactions. "From the fact that each of us constructs a world based on his expectancies, it follows that, to the extent we can influence another person's expectancies, we can affect how he feels, thinks, behaves." (Frank, 1958, p. 216). We can change our focus from illness to wellness through respectful and dignified relationships with persons with HIV and their caregivers. We need to treat caregivers (and patients) as equal partners in our caring relationships. We are there to support them, not judge them.

I offer an example of how a new occupational therapist approached her fears of the unfamiliar when given an opportunity to work with a young homosexual man with HIV. Her conflict was not with the illness, but with his sexual orientation. She walked into his room and sat down near his bed, lowered the bedrails, and offered a cheerful but tenuous greeting. The patient detected her tenuousness. Having become familiar with people's varied reactions to his illness, he asked if she was frightened by HIV. She replied that she was not, but she realized that she was being affected by her lack of knowledge about homosexuality. She expressed concern that this patient was feeling stigmatized because she was not communicating with him about this matter, and she explained to him that she came from an environment that was not open about cultural differences. She replied in a straightforward manner that she had never met an "openly gay" person before and did not know what to say or do. The patient provided the information she needed to help her relax and feel more comfortable. The transformation that took place resulted from this therapist examination of her commitment and service to the patient and of what was needed to provide that service. In this case, what was needed and what was provided were honest communication and conversation about each other's personal, social and cultural values. We often can learn much about ourselves from our patients if we are authentic and honest. Personal transformation is the beginning of the development of honest, authentic and caring relationships.

PROFESSIONAL TRANSFORMATION

I suggest there is a need for transformation in occupational therapy before there can be a universal acknowledgement of the power of occupation in the lives of persons with HIV infection and AIDS. Our profession needs to focus on the art and science of occupation – the examination of occupation in assessment, the use of occupation in treatment, and the scientific study of occupation. Occupation and adaptation, the tools of occupational therapists, can make the difference in a person's quality of living and creation of meaning in the world.

The primary focus of HIV management has been on HIV pathology and medical symptoms because of the urgency to find a vaccine and cure. The social and psychological aspects of HIV have been given greater emphasis only recently. Even with this new emphasis, HIV management has not necessarily included therapy, particularly occupational therapy, services . . . My commitment is that there be universal acknowledgement of the need for occupational therapy services for persons with HIV and AIDS. Such services would not be aligned with the medical model of care but rather would incorporate medical information into a holistic model of care – one that emphasizes occupation.

Occupational therapists do not focus on pathology, but rather on productivity, function and wellness within the value system and on the occupational choices of human beings. Our professional values are grounded in the art and science of occupation. Our clinical reasoning and problem solving are based on thinking in terms of systems and on the integration of the psychosocial, physical and environmental aspects of care in combination with the universal human modality of human touch.

Transformation in the profession, with regard to the HIV pandemic, can occur through an acknowledgement of our history, particularly that which is grounded in Moral Treatment, and a commitment to the fundamental principles of occupational therapy. The purpose of Moral Treatment was to restore patients to improved function and productivity (Bing, 1981). Such occupations as music, literature, physical exercise and particularly, work, were used to develop skills. It was believed that the social environment in which the person was treated should resemble that of a family unit, which incorporated a spiritual dimension. Caregivers used approaches of kindness and consideration, viewed patients as having the ability to change and emphasized a positive prognosis and a strong therapeutic relationship (Bing, 1981). Given the social isolation and loss of family, friends and loved ones resulting from the stigma surrounding HIV, the use of these basic principles of care, which are more aligned with systems thinking than reductionist thinking, can strengthen the integrity, mind and will of persons with HIV and their caregivers.

Occupational therapy can become the role model for the creation of safe and secure environments in which persons with HIV can live, work and function. We need only to believe in the abilities and inherent power of people to change, in the power of occupation, and in the power of ourselves as the catalyst for transformation. Using systems thinking, and committing to the fundamental principles of occupational therapy, as we involve ourselves proactively with persons with HIV, we can strengthen our personal and professional character and integrity and realize the ultimate responsibility of human being to human being.

Yerxa (1967) contributed to this conversation on transformation:

> Philosophically we do not see man as a 'thing' but as a being whose choices allow him to discover and determine his own Being. Our media, our emphasis upon the client's potentials, the necessity for him to act and the mutuality of our relationship with him provide a milieu in which his suffering can be translated into the resolve to become his true self. . . . This is also a time for each of us to determine our own authenticity as professionals. The degree to which we can maintain faith in our profession and still strive to improve it by our own acts, the degree to which we can maintain faith in our clients while becoming involved in the process of helping them will determine the future authenticity of our practice. We are ever becoming. (p. 172)

TRANSFORMATION OF HIV AND AIDS

Thus far in our conversation, I have examined some possibilities for personal and professional transformation that can make a powerful difference in the lives of persons with HIV and their caregivers. Through our personal and professional transformation will come the transformation of HIV. We must also acknowledge, however, other possibilities for transformation, particularly regarding the disease itself.

1. HIV IS NOW CONSIDERED A CHRONIC DISEASE, NOT A TERMINAL DISEASE. The increased life span of people with HIV infection, especially with the advent of life sustaining drugs, is transforming

HIV from a terminal disease to a chronic disease. This includes the many long term survivors of HIV infection. In her analysis of neuroimmuno-modulation, Farber (1989) cited a study that investigated personal attitudes of long term survivors. Among their attitudes and behaviors cited were realistic expectations (e.g., accepting the disease but believing in life), a fighting spirit, a willingness to modify their lifestyles, assertiveness, attention to personal needs, open and honest communication, assumption of responsibility for personal health, and contributions to others (Solomon, Temoshak, O'Leary and Zich, 1987). Occupational therapists can facilitate these attitudes and behaviors to improve the quality of life for persons with chronic HIV infection.

2. POSITIVE AND SUPPORTIVE ATTITUDES OF OCCUPATIONAL THERAPISTS CAN POSITIVELY INFLUENCE THE STATE OF HEALTH OF PEOPLE WITH HIV. Persons with HIV are devastated physically, psychologically and spiritually and most likely have encountered prejudice and discrimination before and after their diagnosis of HIV. We have an opportunity to support people with HIV through nonjudgmental, positive approaches to life and living and to use our power as a catalyst for transformation. We can provide hope and meaning to patients through adaptation, occupation, and a positive spirit without providing false hope for a cure.

3. STEREOTYPES SHOULD BE AVOIDED. Human beings often have a preexisting interpretation of each other, of situations, and of how things ought to be. In caring for patients with HIV infection, therapists must avoid any preexisting interpretations of what gay persons should look like or what their interests should be, how an intravenous drug user usually responds to others, or even what a person with HIV infection should present clinically. Stereotyping is much like judging others, and it creates boxes, or categories, in which patients are placed. Patients, as well, may have a stereotype of who we are as health care providers, on the basis of their positive and negative experiences with the health care system. Transformation begins when we see each other as unique and with a special contribution to make. The inclusion of life-style and subcultural (e.g., gay, bisexual, intravenous drug user) needs in our HIV assessments and treatments shows our respect for the person's individuality.

4. NO ONE PERSON OR GROUP OF PERSONS IS TO BLAME FOR HIV. HIV does not discriminate — people do. The discoverers of HIV, Gallo and Montagnier (1988), believed that the virus had existed in small, isolated groups of people in central Africa or elsewhere for years. Because these groups had little contact with the outside world, HIV stayed

within the groups. As the way of life changed in central Africa, the pattern of transmission most likely was affected. Migration from remote areas to urban centers increased, sexual mores changed and blood transfusions became more common (Gallo and Montagnier, 1988). "Once a pool of infected people had been established, transport networks and the generalized exchange of blood products would have carried it to every corner of the world" (p. 47). The reality is: HIV Is here and must be dealt with.

5. HUMAN TOUCH IS BOTH IMPORTANT AND NECESSARY. Universal precautions to benefit the patient and ourselves have been implemented world-wide (U.S. Department of Health and Human Services, 1988). It is vital that we give ourselves and our patients and their caregivers permission to experience connectedness through touch. It is feasible, without gloves, to hug, hold and touch HIV-infected persons when precautions are unnecessary (e.g., when the therapist is not at risk for exposure to blood and body fluids). Huss (1976) stated: "Touching involves risk . . . If we are not in tune with ourselves and the one we touch, it may be inappropriate. However, non-touch may be just as devastating at a time when words are insufficient or cannot be processed appropriately because of disintegration of the individual" (p. 305).

6. A VIEW OF AIDS AS A CONVERSATION. A shift in thinking, or a transformation, can occur most easily when we think of AIDS in terms of a conversation, that is, not something that simply IS a certain way but, rather, something that can be altered by the way in which we speak or think about it. We as occupational therapists can transform the conversation called AIDS through our personal and professional transformation and through our commitment to the conversation called the art and science of occupational therapy.

THE FUTURE

Future vaccines and strategies will alter the course of the HIV pandemic and increase the number of long term survivors. Recent research has demonstrated the effectiveness of an HIV vaccine in monkeys, which is "the first truly promising step toward creating a human AIDS vaccine (Specter, 1989, pp. 1, 12). Until there is a cure, knowledge and education are the best strategies to combat this disease.

Occupational therapy is on the forefront of transforming the conversation about HIV and AIDS. Our belief in occupation and in the possibilities for human beings for productive living will support us. Questions for us to examine, given the possibilities for HIV-infected children and adults living long and full lives, include the following:

1. What will the role of occupational therapy be for the chronic HIV patient throughout a normal lifespan? How can occupational therapy be effective in developing normalized occupational roles such as student, player and friend for HIV infected children who reach adulthood?
2. What are the current and future mental health problems of persons with HIV and their caregivers and what will occupational therapy's role be in meeting the current and future needs of this population?
3. What will the clinical picture be of children with HIV, on permanent drug treatments, who become workers in society? Will special adaptations be needed? What will be the special mental health problems of these children, if any, related directly to the stigma of HIV infection? Will occupational therapy be called on to make a difference?
4. How can occupational therapists develop adaptive environments along the developmental continuum to promote adaptive occupational behaviors for long term survivors of HIV?
5. Can occupational therapy be a vital service in industries that have HIV infected persons who wish to maintain their worker roles? How can occupational therapy promote continued productivity and well being in the workplace despite the stigma and chronic illness that disrupts habits, roles and skills?
6. How can occupational therapy make a significant contribution in minority communities in which the prevalence of HIV is increasing? What program development skills can we offer?
7. What types of creative wellness programs can occupational therapists develop for children and adults with HIV and their caregivers?
8. What role will occupational therapy play in developing family-centered care for adults and children with HIV infection and AIDS?
9. What role will occupational therapy play in addressing the special needs of women affected by HIV (e.g., women who themselves have HIV infection or who are caring for others with HIV infection)? What occupational therapy services are necessary to support the development and maintenance of these occupational roles?

These are a few of the many questions occupational therapists are going to face. We can begin our transformation now or allow the fear of risk taking to stop us.

We are all afraid—for our confidence, for the future, for the world. That is the nature of human imagination. Yet every man, every civilization, has gone forward because of its engagement with what it has set itself out to do. The personal commitment of a man to his skills, the intellectual commitment and the emotional commitment working together, has made the Ascent of Man. (Bronowski, 1973, p. 432)

Regarding the AIDS epidemic, by aligning with this personal, intellectual and emotional commitment, occupational therapy will make a difference on a societal and global level. It is our opportunity for transformation.

REFERENCES

Bing, R. (1981). Eleanor Clarke Slagle Lectureship—1981—Occupational therapy revisited: A paraphrastic journey. *American Journal of Occupational Therapy*, 35, 499-518.
Bronowski, J. (1973). *The ascent of man*. Boston: Little, Brown.
Farber, S.D. (1989). 1989 Eleanor Clarke Slagle Lecture—Neuroscience and occupational therapy: Vital connections. *American Journal of Occupational Therapy*, 43, 637-646.
Ferguson, M. (1980). *The aquarian conspiracy*. Los Angeles: J.P. Tarcher.
Frank, J.D. (1958). The therapeutic use of self. *American Journal of Occupational Therapy*, 12, 215-225.
Gallo, R.C. and Montagnier, L. (1988, October). AIDS in 1988. *Scientific American*, pp. 40-48.
Huss, A.J. (1977). 1976 Eleanor Clarke Slagle Lecture—Touch with care or a caring touch? *American Journal of Occupational Therapy*, 31, 11-18.
Institute of Medicine. (1988). *Confronting AIDS: Update 1988*. Washington, DC: National Academy Press.
May, R. (1975). *The courage to create*. New York: W.W. Norton.
Specter, M. (1989, December 8). AIDS vaccine proves effective in monkeys. *Washington Post*, pp. 1,12.
Yerxa, E.J. (1967). 1966 Eleanor Clarke Slagle Lecture—Authentic occupational therapy. *American Journal of Occupational Therapy*, 21, 1-9.

Values and Life Goals: Clinical Interventions for People with AIDS

Judith K. Williams, MSW, LCSW

SUMMARY. This article will address the development of strategies and therapeutic interventions which may be used to help PWAs (people with AIDS) cope with the illness and assist them in the re-evaluation of life goals and changes in values from those of the living to those of the dying. Clinical interventions designed to empower PWAs to take control of their lives and to play an active part in their medical care are outlined.

INTRODUCTION

Acquired immune deficiency syndrome (AIDS) has had a major impact on the lives of those who are diagnosed with the disease, their friends and families, their caregivers, and their communities. Society has been slow to accept the severity and extent of the AIDS epidemic. Many lives have been changed by this disease and through adversity, pain, physical and mental suffering and loss, some significant growth has occurred. Values, life goals, priorities and relationships have been altered and, in many cases, a sense of commitment, altruism, and self confidence has emerged. In daily contacts with people with AIDS (PWAs), with their friends and families and with medical professionals who work with PWAs, their determination to fight the illness and to control the opportunistic infections which accompany it has been clearly evident. In the midst of tragedy and

Judith K. Williams is Clinical Social Worker/Psychotherapist at the National Institutes of Health in Bethesda, Maryland. She works with patients at the National Institute of Allergy and Infectious Diseases and is an active member of the multidisciplinary HIV program of the institute. Ms. Williams is associated with the Whitman-Walker Clinic of Washington, D.C., where she is a pro bono therapist.

55

grief PWAs have re-examined their priorities and made contributions in finding treatments for AIDS as well as other diseases.

BACKGROUND

AIDS was first described in 1979. However, many health care facilities did not diagnose their first patients until 1982 or 1983. In the early years the disease was often referred to as "The Gay Plague" and it was seen by some as a punishment meted out for the sexual practices of homosexuals. Later it became clear that while the disease was spread through the Gay community by unprotected anal intercourse, it was also spreading through the heterosexual Haitian community. It was also found among intravenous drug users and infected hemophiliacs and others who received transfusions or blood products contaminated with the virus (Cassens, 1985).

The disease affects the immune system of the body and the patient becomes the target of many opportunistic infections (Dimond, 1989). These infections include pneumocystis pneumonia carinii (PCP), Kaposi's sarcoma (KS), cytomegalovirus (CMV) and numerous other fungal and viral infections. In the early years medical science had little to offer the AIDS patient who typically was encountered in a hospital emergency room feverish, emaciated, coughing with the pneumonia which we now know is caused by pneumocystis carinii, and covered by the distinctive purple blotches of Kaposi's sarcoma. With recent advances, AIDS is no longer the acute terminal disease of the early 1980s but a chronic terminal illness. As advances are made in treating the symptoms of the disease and the opportunistic infections which develop due to the failure of the patient's immune system to fight infection, many patients live longer with an improved quality of life.

PSYCHOSOCIAL PROBLEMS

In addition to the physical manifestations of AIDS, PWAs present with psychosocial problems. Among these problems are:

1. Coping with a life threatening illness.
2. Fear of death, of being alone and of the illness and its course.
3. Guilt over acquiring the disease and perhaps infecting others, guilt over leaving loved ones behind with no caregiver and guilt caused by the stigma society places on those suffering from a sexually transmitted disease.

4. Anger at being infected with the disease and at those who may have transmitted the disease.

Nearly all patients are depressed at some point in the course of the illness (Kubler-Ross, 1987). Most suffer from shock when they first learn they are infected, and support, empathy and honest counseling are crucial at this time. The reality of the diagnosis often precipitates suicidal ideation. Skilled intervention can help the patient deal with the crisis he or she faces and provide a good start in making changes which will help throughout the course of the disease.

CRISIS INTERVENTION THERAPY

When the diagnosis of HIV infection is made, a psychological crisis often develops. Usually the person, who is being tested, has hoped and prayed that the test will be negative, while fearing and suspecting that it will be positive. A positive diagnosis initiates feelings of shock, fear, anger and loss of control which call for immediate and skilled therapeutic intervention. It is important that counseling be available at this crucial time and that the PWA receive support and an opportunity to ventilate feelings in a safe and confidential atmosphere.

The Chinese characters for the word crisis are danger and opportunity. At the time of crisis PWAs are often able to make important changes which will improve their ability to cope with the diagnosis. Such changes include a shift or alteration in lifestyle and planning for adaptive initiatives in the areas of employment, education and life goals. Therapists can help the client respond positively to this opportunity for change and growth. Crisis intervention therapy is well suited to the medical setting and the clinical skills acquired through work with patients suffering from cancer, cardiac problems and other chronic and acute illnesses prepare the clinician for working with the PWA.

REASSESSMENT OF VALUES

Recently announced results of research conducted at the National Institute of Allergy and Infectious Disease (NIAID) indicate that there is significant delay of the symptoms associated with AIDS (Fauci, 1989) by those who began early treatment with AZT (zidovudine). This is good news for those who test positive for HIV, as it lengthens the time that they remain well and able to function independently. This development provides additional time for reassessing values, for setting long term goals and mapping out ways to reach those goals.

Often a therapy assignment which helps PWAs is a listing of their personal values. What does the PWA value in life? Values are developed from childhood and the PWA will often reflect on the values of his family, community or religion. The reality of the diagnosis of HIV infection may cause clients to modify their values. Ambition to get ahead in ones career, to impress others and to be accepted by the "in crowd" are very often mediated by the impact of the infection. PWAs begin to take control of their lives and do what they really want to do, not what others want or expect them to do (Milan & Ross, 1987). PWAs may renew their religious ties or choose spiritual guidance from a new source. Many begin to take care of their health for the first time in their lives. They become knowledgeable about diet, exercise and stress reduction techniques. Less emphasis is placed on what others think and more emphasis on self improvement and self care. Altruism (a concern for the disadvantaged, for society and for the oppressed), personal honesty, sensitivity to others and to the environment are common values listed by PWAs.

One patient, after coping with the initial shock of finding that he was HIV positive, decided to return to school and study computers. He had a plan to combine his training and talent in design with computer skills and start a business out of his home. He thought that he would be able to do this work even if he did eventually become too ill to go out to a job. He also wanted to be able to set his own work schedule, thus enabling him to keep doctor's appointments and help out at a community action committee office without affecting his work.

This patient was seen recently, still feeling quite well nearly two years after his diagnosis. He has finished his courses and is starting to get referrals for his company. He thinks that he would still be working as a waiter with only a dream of going back to school and starting a business if he had not been shocked into action by the diagnosis of HIV infection. He joked about our first meeting just after his test results were known. He had asked at that time, in complete seriousness, whether he should start making funeral plans. He was initially so terrified and so completely at a loss that he felt his life was over. Hearing the facts and getting support to take control of his situation was very important to him.

The patient, who was seen for supportive task oriented psychotherapy, spent several weeks sorting through his hopes and dreams and developing a list of goals and priorities. At first he did not want to tell anyone about his positive test; then he went through a period of telling everyone (even those who did not need to know and those who used this information against him). Finally he came to deal with the reality of the positive test and, accepting this reality, he was able to go forward with his life and plans. He retained his true friends, lost those who really did not care about him or who were too judgemental to accept him and his condition, and made many new friends at school and in the community action committee where he gives help and support to others in need (Williams, 1989).

LIFE REVIEW

We see in PWAs the same need to examine their lives and evaluate their contributions that Robert N. Butler, MD so clearly explained as "Life Review," a task of the elderly who were nearing death (Butler, 1975) However, PWAs are much younger, usually between 25-45 years of age, compared to those in their seventies and eighties as described by Butler. Nevertheless it is just as important that PWAs gain a sense of their impact upon society. These contributions may be great or small, but are significant to the PWA. One patient described the dinner parties he planned, the food he cooked and the pleasure his friends derived from these special social functions as an example of the contribution he had made on a regular basis.

Another PWA devoted many hours as a caregiver for a friend who died of AIDS some time ago. He enabled his friend to remain at home, surrounded by the things he loved, until his death. Helping others, teaching, creating, writing, lobbying are examples of the valuable tasks performed by PWAS. These contributions to others offer psychic support to the dying PWA. The PWA must be able to say, "My life was worthwhile; I did some good things and hopefully I will be able to do even more of value before I die."

PWAs want to feel self worth and experience self esteem, otherwise they will experience the despair often seen in the elderly (Erikson, 1950). Despair is present when the PWA says "I might as well die and get it over with—I've never done anything worthwhile anyway." This type of statement is a call for help.

The experience of one very ill patient being treated for PCP (pneumocystis carnii pneumonia) illustrates this despair. He had been rejected by his parents some years earlier due to his homosexuality. He was derided and taunted by his alcoholic sister and had only the support of his brother to sustain him at home. His lover of many years had died about a year earlier from complications of AIDS. It was a cold dreary February and the patient had been hospitalized for several weeks. He was depressed and stated that he wished his struggle against AIDS would soon be over.

In daily bedside sessions with this patient, it emerged that he was a gardener. He always loved plants and kept his neighbors and friends supplied with flowers and vegatables when he had been well. The following day when the patient was given seed catalogues, he was delighted and pored over the pictures and descriptions of the plants. He became markedly more alert and verbal with patients and staff. He discussed planting, gardens of the past and plans for spring planting. He ordered seeds, started seeds under a small growlight, diagrammed his garden plot and at last was able to see that he had a talent and had made a contribution to others through his gardening skills. He supplied many staff members with seedlings which are still growing in their gardens (Simmons-Alling, 1984). This patient was discharged from the hospital and lived for some years with a renewed sense of self worth and of self esteem. Every PWA has worth and even though young, has affected the lives of others. It is the task of the therapist to help patients identify their contributions, through discovery of their talents and skills (Kushner, 1981).

FAMILY ISSUES

People with terminal illnesses often want to resolve inter- personal problems and to heal old wounds. PWAs may be estranged from their biological families due to lifestyle conflicts. Since PWAs are often young they may not have reached a rapprochement with their parents which follows the separation of young adults from their homes of origin. There may also be unresolved problems stemming from the sexual orientation of the son or daughter, which has not been brought into the open and discussed with the parents (Govoni, 1988).

Rifts in the family may have existed for some years, and the PWA may want to heal them before death. In these cases siblings can often play the role of mediator by advocating for the understanding and acceptance of the parents (Johnson, 1987).

In one case a young PWA regretted the lack of contact he had with his elderly father. His father was now old and ill with a heart condition. The PWA wanted to spend a Christmas with his father and asked his sister and the family priest to help intervene on his behalf with his father. Interestingly the PWA's father was also anxious to put aside the anger and quarrels of the past.

The PWA was able to spend an enjoyable Christmas with his father and sister in the family home. He returned to his own home in good spirits with peace of mind from the reconciliation with his father and pleased that he had been able to tell his father how much he loved and respected him. The father reportedly also found satisfaction in accepting his son again and in telling him of his pride in the son's many accomplishments. Ironically the father died shortly before the New Year and the PWA died on New Year's day. However both were at peace with each other and both had resolved the problems which had been bothering them about their relationship.

SEXUALITY AND STIGMA

There are times when the parents remain rigid and unaccepting. They may feel guilt at their own inadequacies in dealing with sexuality and see their child's sexual choices as reflections on their parenting and often as their failure to instill their religious and social beliefs in an effective manner. There is in our society a lack of knowledge of human sexuality and a perception that there is only one accepted way to deal with sexual urges (i.e., through marriage and heterosexual intercourse) (DeCecco, 1984).

Little education is available concerning alternative sexual preferences and sexual fulfillment. Seldom discussed is the fact that many men and women are sexually repressed and never receive fulfillment through socially accepted sexual practice. Those who do not conform to the societal norms are viewed as abnormal and often treated as sexual deviants (Cohen & Weisman, 1986).

The stigma of the sexually transmitted disease which is placed upon the PWA by society is not a new development with this disease. Susan Sontag (1989) reviews the historical labelling of diseases and makes it clear why AIDS has been called a plague. She finds that plagues are invariably regarded as judgments on society, and the metaphoric inflation of AIDS into such a judgment also accustoms people to the inevitability of global spread.

Since AIDS is primarily sexually transmitted it is even more apt to be viewed as punishment for evil, immorality and/or obscene behavior. Others, who were infected by blood products, in utero or by needle pricks are viewed by society as innocent victims of the evil ways of others. Perhaps the historical case of syphilis and its spread most nearly approaches the disapprobation society attaches to AIDS (Gilman, 1988). Syphilis was blamed on prostitutes and the men who were tempted by them were seen as weak, but victimized by the licentious behavior of these evil women (Sontag, 1977). AIDS and syphilis are comparable not only in terms of society's attitudes toward the victims but, with the recent medical advances that have made AIDS more of a chronic and less of an acute disease, they have become epidemiologically more comparable.

The PWA and the therapist must constantly battle the social stigma and attempt to educate the public. This is an onerous task for a person fighting for wellness in the face of severe viral infection and a poorly functioning immune system. It is also a challenge for those professions, who, on the basis of ethics and insight, reject judgmental pronouncements as being representative of guilt, fear and ignorance.

One of the major psychological problems which profoundly affects PWAs is reactive depression. Certainly everyone can understand the reasons a person would feel depressed upon receiving the diagnosis of AIDS. AIDS is a progressive disease and, at this time, it is a terminal process. The prognosis is death. However, as noted previously, the length of time in which the PWA can expect to live with a good quality of life is increasing as new treatments are discovered. The PWA is faced with riding the rollercoaster of chronic illness with its peaks of wellness and dips into the troughs of illness.

CATHARSIS IS THERAPEUTIC

The scheduled short hospitalization to treat one opportunistic infection can extend as complications set in and other infections occur. The PWA cannot and must not be expected to be forever stoic and cheerful. Medical staff, friends and family must allow the PWA to get in touch with feelings and be allowed to feel sad, angry and frustrated. The idea that the terminally ill must be always jolly and smiling must be abandoned. Sometimes it is necessary to step back and realize that the falsely cheerful facade is for the benefit of others and may actually be detrimental to the PWA.

Often PWAs come to the social worker's office to cry, express their anger or to ventilate their frustrations with this very complicated and tough disease. They feel a safety in the therapeutic relationship which allows them to bring their feelings to the surface and then out into the open. They realize that they will not be judged weak, lacking in strength or as having given up but rather as having an opportunity to get the terrible weight of their repressed feelings off of their hearts and minds. This venting of emotions is called catharsis. Often clients leave a therapy session with the feelings stated by one PWA, "I feel like a heavy load has been taken off of my shoulders and a weight lifted from my heart. Now I have the confidence to fight this disease with renewed energy."

A young mother who developed AIDS after receiving a pint of blood following surgery was afraid to let her anger and sadness surface. "What good will it do to give in to these feelings?" she said. "I must take one day at a time and keep my emotions controlled or I might start crying and never stop." Unfortunately, this PWAs family would not let her talk about her illness or to think about the future. They tried to deny the reality of the disease by refusing to acknowledge it. This denial is a defense mechanism developed to protect one from psychological pain.

In the case of this young woman the inability to ventilate her feelings led to bizarre reactions to illness. She felt that to cry and scream due to pain would be acceptable. Her family could understand reactions to acute pain, but could not accept reactions to psychic pain. Therefore this woman over-reacted to any medical procedure which caused even the slightest pain. To prick a finger for a drop of blood, to take a normal blood pressure reading or to receive an injection brought about a severe reaction. The patient would scream, cry and thrash about in her bed for a period of time. Following these outbursts the patient reported that she felt better.

After some time and after gaining trust in the therapist, the patient was able to report that she was unable to keep her feelings inside any longer. To save her family the pain of dealing with her illness and prognosis, she would experience emotional outbursts to vent some of the anger and deep emotions she felt. She was able to see that this way of coping with her feelings was not productive and began to use therapy sessions as a time of ventilation and catharsis. The patient was able to begin to discuss her true feelings without fear of losing control. The fear of sinking into a morass of self pity and depression was unfounded and had kept this patient from developing plans and coping skills at an earlier phase of her illness.

EFFECTS OF STRESS

Studies showing the deleterious effect of stress on the functioning of the immune system are accepted now by medical professionals. Unfortunately these findings appear not to be widely understood by the general public. There seems to be little awareness of the extent to which stress caused by suppressed feelings of anxiety, depression, anger and confusion can interfere with the body's ability to combat infection (Frierson & Lippman, 1987).

The POMS-LASA (profile of mood states combined with a linear analogue self assessment questionaire) which has been applied so effectively to cancer patients (Sutherland, Lockwood & Cunningham, 1989) is relevant and could be applied just as effectively to PWAs. This testing allows the clinician to discover the level of coping skills available to the patient and will give a clearer picture of the specific problem areas to be worked on in therapy sessions. Due to socialization, and often to spare others from pain, terminally ill patients may bury their feelings (Felton, Revenson & Hinrichsen, 1984). It is difficult to dissuade a well meaning parent or lover that keeping a "stiff upper lip" may not be helping the PWA and in fact may be slowing his recovery from infection (Goldberg & Tull, 1983).

Another very difficult problem faced by PWAs is suicidal ideation. We know that suicidal ideation is often found among the chronically and terminally ill (Kubler-Ross, 1969). Certainly a person faced with the prognosis of death might think about prematurely ending his life to save himself and his family from pain. However, many people deny that they have ever thought about suicide, and they deny thinking about death as such thoughts are not widely acceptable in our society (Dilley & Ochitill, 1985). It is healthy for those who are facing death to think about it to some extent. Morbid preoccupation with death is a far cry from thinking and talking about what lies ahead and how death might come. Too often PWAs are not allowed to talk about their views of death or to ask questions about how they might die (Deucher, 1984). They should not be judged as psychotic just because they think about death and perhaps taking their own lives to end pain and suffering.

It is important for them to know that there are effective pain medications which can remove the specter of unbearable pain from them as death nears. Often a straight forward explanation of how they will be kept comfortable and pain free at the end of their lives removes the need for them to focus on methods of suicide (Christ, Wiener & Moynihan, 1986).

Fear of the unknown and fear of loss of control often leads a patient to consider taking his own life. A PWA who is given information and allowed to make decisions about a course of treatment and about any heroic measures to be taken if confronted with a critical illness feels empowered. This empowerment and renewed sense of self control raises self worth and self esteem. Suicidal plans can be replaced by confidence in those who will carry out instructions if the PWA becomes too impaired mentally and physically to make decisions about life or death.

Most hospitals and clinics now provide information about living wills and designated powers of attorney, which enable a PWA to choose a friend or relative to make necessary medical decisions. Planning for death often makes life more bearable and a PWA can focus on living knowing that dying is taken care of by those in whom one has trust. This control of the future is empowering and helps the PWA, close associates and family cope with whatever lies ahead.

CONCLUSION

AIDS has made a great impact on our society, and those who have contracted the disease have done much to educate others about methods of coping with chronic illness and living with dying. They have helped us gain strength and learn lessons about how human beings can rise above adversity and attain new levels of self-sacrifice and altruism through contact with those who are devoted to finding answers to control and someday conquer this disease. The values and goals which have been transformed through hard work and planning offer inspiration to those working within the medical field and those in society at large who have an opportunity to see progress with minds unclouded by prejudice and ignorance.

QUESTIONS

1. *What is the therapeutic modality usually applicable to the period following the initial diagnosis of HIV infection?*
2. *What is the strategy described by the gerontologist, Dr. Robert N. Butler, to help the elderly gain self esteem?*
3. *What is the type of depression often seen in PWAs as they try to cope with their disease.*
4. *What other sexually transmitted disease was stigmatized by society in the Victorian period?*
5. *What are the legal documents which PWAs can use to make provisions for their medical treatment when they are seriously ill?*

ANSWERS

1. Crisis intervention therapy is well suited to the period of initial diagnosis as it offers an opportunity for change and adaptation.
2. Dr. Robert N. Butler described "Life Review" as a useful tool in providing the aged a way to document their worth and support their egos as they near death.
3. PWA's often develop reactive depression. This depression is not marked by the symptoms of sleep disturbance, weight loss, withdrawal and suicidal ideation found in clinical depression. The therapist must carefully monitor for signals of a clinical depression.
4. Syphilis was viewed as a stigma due to its sexual transmission.
5. Living wills and designated powers of attorney enable the PWA to

have some input into his medical cares and any heroic measures taken when he is nearing death.

REFERENCES

Altman, D., (1986). *AIDS in the mind of America*. New York: Anchor Press.
Buscaglia, Leo, (1982). *Living, loving and learning*. New York: Holt, Rinehart and Winston.
Butler, Robert N., (1975). *Why survive? : Being old in America*. New York: Harper and Roe.
Cassens, B.J., (1985). Social consequences of acquired immunodeficiency syndrome. *Annals of Internal Medicine. 103*(11). 761-771.
Christ, G.H., Wiener, L.S. & Moynihan, R.T., (1986). Psychosocial issues in AIDS. *Psychiatric Annals. 16*(3). 173-179.
Cohen, M.A. & Weisman, H.W., (1986). A biopsychosocial approach to AIDS. *Psychosomatics. 27*(4). 245-249.
Coleman, E., (1982). Developmental stages of the coming out process. In J. Gonsiorek (Ed.). *Homosexuality and Psychotherapy*. New York: Haworth Press.
DeCecco, J.P.(Ed.)., (1984). *Homophobia: An Overview*. New York: Haworth Press.
Deucher, N., (1984). AIDS in New York City with particular reference to the psycho-social aspects. *British Journal of Psychiatry. 145*. 612-619.
Dilley, J.W., & Ochitill, H.N., (1985). Findings in psychiatric consultations with patients with acquired immune deficiency syndrome. *American Journal of Psychiatry. 142*:1. 82-85.
Dimond, P.F., (1989). AIDS — associated opportunistic infections pose diagnostic dilemmas. *Diagnostics and Clinical Testing. 27*:6. 25-27.
Erikson, E.H., (1950). *Identity and the life cycle*. New York: International Universities Press.
Erikson, E.H., (1950). Generativity and ego integrity. In B.L. Neugarten (Ed.) *Middle age and aging*. Chicago: University of Chicago Press.
Fauci, A., (1989). National Institute of Allergy and Infectious Disease press release. National Institutes of Health Record. Bethesda: National Institutes of Health Press.
Felton, B.J., Revenson, T.A., and Hinrichsen, (1984). Coping with chronic illness: controllability and the influence of coping strategies on psychological adjustment. *Journal of Consulting and Clinical Psychology. 52*. 343-353.
Frierson, R.L., & Lippmann, S.B., (1987). Stresses on physicians treating AIDS. *American Family Practitioner. 35*:6. 153-159.
Gilman, S.L., (1988) AIDS and syphilis: The iconography of disease. In D. Crimp (Ed.). *AIDS: Cultural analysis, cultural activism*. Cambridge, Massachusetts: The MIT Press.

Goldberg, R.J. and Tull, R.M., (1983). *The psychological dimensions of cancer.* New York: Free Press.

Govoni, L.A., (1988) Psychological issues of AIDs in the nursing care of homosexual men and their significant others. *Nursing Clinics of North America.* 23:4.

Johnson, S., (1987). AIDS psychological stresses on the family. *Psychosomatics.* 28:2. 65-68.

Kubler-Ross, E., (1987). *AIDS: The ultimate challenge.* New York: MacMillan.

Kubler-Ross, E., (1969). *On Death and Dying.* New York: MacMillan.

Kushner, H.S., (1981). *When Bad Things Happen to Good People.* New York: Avon Books.

Milan, G. and Ross, M.W., (1987). AIDS and gay youth: attitudes and lifestyle modifications in young male homosexuals. *Community Health Studies.* 11:1. 50-53.

Morin, S.F., & Malyon, A.K., (1987). Meeting psychological needs in the AIDS crisis. B.C. Moffatt, & J. Spiegal (Eds.). *AIDS: A Self-Care Manual.* Santa Monica, California: IBS Press.

Simmons-Alling, S., (1984). AIDS: psychosocial needs of the health care worker. *Topics in Clinical Nursing.* 6:2. 31-37.

Sontag, S., (1977). *Illness as Metaphor.* New York: Farrar, Strause and Giroux.

Sontag, S., (1988). *AIDS and Its Metaphors.* New York: Farrar, Strause and Giroux.

Sutherland, H.J., Lockwood, G.A., & Cunningham, A.J., (1989). A simple, rapid method for assessing psychological distress in cancer patients: Evidence for validity for linear analog scales. *Journal of Psychosocial Oncology.* 7:1/2.

Williams, M.J., (1989). Gay men as "buddies" to persons living with AIDS and ARC. *Smith College Social Work Journal.* 2.

Cultural Considerations
in the Treatment
of Persons with AIDS

Marjorie E. Scaffa, PhD (Cand.), MS, OTR/L
Donna A. Davis, MPH

SUMMARY. The impact of AIDS has been most notable in three subpopulations in the United States: the gay community, intravenous drug abusers and minority groups, particularly Blacks and Hispanics. Little information is available on the cultural considerations which are relevant in the treatment of these individuals. This article describes basic principles of cross-cultural analysis, explores individual aspects of AIDS in these populations and discusses the implications for health care providers.

INTRODUCTION

Of the health care dilemmas that the medical community faces today, none has as far-reaching and severe a potential impact on the international community as Acquired Immunodeficiency Syndrome, (AIDS). An extensive body of literature exists in nearly all social and clinical sciences, as the effects of the disease have social, medical, ethical, psychological and moral implications. As with many other disease entities, there is a large number of resources available to assist health professionals in dealing with the scientific and clinical aspects of the disease, but much less information on the cultural considerations in the prevention and treatment of AIDS.

Marjorie E. Scaffa is Occupational Therapist and PhD candidate and Instructor in the Department of Health Education at the University of Maryland, College Park, MD 20742.

Donna A. Davis is a doctoral student and Graduate Assistant in the Department of Health Education at the University of Maryland, College Park, MD 20742.

69

An understanding of the factors which impact on health behavior is basic in the development of any prevention or treatment plan. This understanding is even more essential when dealing with members of a subculture of the general population, since certain cultural aspects can significantly facilitate or impede efforts toward successful treatment. Especially important in this discussion are the knowledge, attitudes, beliefs, values, roles and lifestyle that a patient brings to the clinical situation. These factors provide the rationale or motivation for behavior and impact communication strategies in helping relationships.

In the mainstream health care system, cultural insensitivity can lead to institutional policies that are contrary to the values of specific groups; misunderstandings between providers and patients due to differences in expectations, cultural norms and communication styles; and the development of distrust of the health care system by cultural groups arising out of a series of negative experiences. It is therefore very important for each of us to examine our own values, expectations, assumptions and practices and consider how these influence and impact on our interactions with individuals from cultural groups other than our own.

Currently, in the United States, there are three important subpopulations which have been most severely affected by the HIV epidemic, the homosexual/bisexual community, intravenous drug abusers and minority populations, particularly Blacks and Hispanics. This chapter will (1) describe basic principles which are applicable in cross-cultural analysis; (2) review the extent of the problem in various sub-populations; (3) explore the cultural considerations of AIDS in these populations and (4) discuss the implications for health care providers. For the purposes of this article, the term AIDS will include persons in all stages of HIV infection.

BASIC PRINCIPLES

Culture, for the purposes of this article, is defined by the authors as a set of factors or ways of living that describe and differentiate a group of human beings and is transmitted from generation to generation. Culture can include superficial and obvious factors, such as diet, dress and music, and more complex phenomena, such as the values, assumptions, priorities and relationships to which a social group ascribes.

The cultural descriptions of minorities, intravenous drug abusers and homosexuals that follow are based on several assumptions (Foster, 1971; Wright, 1984):

1. not all descriptions of a sub-population are applicable to all members of that sub-population in all situations;
2. the differences *between* cultures and subgroups of those cultures are greater than the differences *within* culture and subgroups of those cultures;
3. the cultural considerations presented here are not intended to be exhaustive; and
4. philosophical inquiry into cultural considerations does not rely solely on published literature for validity but also on "stories, oral tradition, ritual, social institutions and so forth as purveyors of thought" (Wright, 1984, p. 51).

The recognition of these basic principles is necessary for health care providers to avoid bias, prejudice and stereotyping of cultural sub-populations.

AIDS AND MINORITIES

The problem of AIDS has had a profound impact upon the Black and Hispanic communities in the United States. Although 26% of AIDS cases are among Blacks, Blacks constitute only 12% of the population of the United States. Similarly, Hispanics make up approximately 6% of the United States' population and 14% of the AIDS cases (JAMA, 1989).

Black Americans

The Black population totals approximately 26.5 million persons, constituting the largest minority in the United States. The majority of Blacks live in urban areas and as is true with other minority populations, Blacks are not homogeneous as a group. Blacks exhibit great variation in educational levels, socioeconomic status, and religion (Department of Health and Human Services, 1985). In spite of this diversity, some cultural similarities are evident and these characteristics can have profound influences on health beliefs, sources of health information, communication in health care relationships and the acceptance of health care.

Traditional Health Beliefs

Studies of the prevalence of folk or traditional health beliefs in the Black population can provide interesting information about the attitudes of Blacks towards AIDS. Snow (1983) reviewed some traditional health beliefs and practices among lower class Black Americans, especially those who had been socialized in the rural South or who maintained kinship ties in the South, or both. Perceptions of many events, including illness, are closely related to religious beliefs and events are generally classified as "natural" or "unnatural." Studies from the fields of sociology and anthropology indicate that many lower class Black Americans view the world as a dangerous, unpredictable place where the most sensible course of action is to always be "on guard."

Natural events are those which are consistent with God's intentions for the world. They are harmonious with nature and, to a large extent, predictable. Natural illnesses occur when the source of the problem is natural, for example, impurities in the air, food or water which may cause illness. Unnatural illnesses occur when someone has done something so serious that God withdraws his protection and allows evil influences to afflict an individual. Belief in witchcraft is common among Haitians, Trinidadians and Black Americans, as well as in other cultural groups (Snow, 1974).

Other Influencing Factors

One way to understand a society is to study its axiology, or what is most valued among the members of that culture. According to Nichols (1988) and Menkiti (1984), relationships have the highest value in the Black American culture. In the "pure" Africanized world view, people and the phenomenal world are indistinct; people feel, experience, internalize and personalize the world around them (Dixon, 1976).

Differences in cultural expectations and values are frequently the cause of misunderstandings in the health care arena. Dixon (1976) postulates that there are significant differences between African-American and Euro-American values, orientation toward human/nature relations, time and activity. For example, Euro-Americans view time as a series of discrete moments which can be utilized as a commodity. In this society "time is money" and preplanning and scheduling are fundamental to success. In the Afro-American culture time is experienced and felt and therefore scheduling and preplanning are not as important as continuing to respond to the events one is experiencing in the here and now. Dixon (1976) quotes an example of this phenomenon in his description of a mental health clinic in Watts that was facing 80% no-show rates for pre-arranged counseling appointments. Research showed that Afro-American patients would appear as "walk-ins" because they used clinic visits only when they needed help. For them "saving up" their feelings for some future appointment date was irrational and illogical. When patients were asked to phone for an appointment on the day a felt-need arose, the show rate rose to 90%.

Perhaps because of limited access to the mainstream health care system in the past, Blacks tend to be skeptical and have negative impressions of medical care (Cope, 1985). For the same reason, members of the Black family, particularly the extended family, have had important roles as caretakers and counselors.

Implications for Health Care Providers

For many Black Americans, beliefs about illness and the blood may partially explain the apparent denial of the seriousness of positive HIV status in the population. When someone believes that blood responds directly to various internal and external stimuli, it may be difficult to grasp the concept of a long-term, continuous disease state. Health care professionals who are aware of these beliefs can address them by inquiring of patients about their health beliefs and correcting misconceptions early on and throughout the treatment process.

A Southern tradition of "I can do" is part of the history of many Black Americans (Mays and Cochran, 1987). This sense of independence may make it difficult to accept and develop appropriately dependent relationships with people outside the family or community networks. This is especially true when dealing with Black males, who typically associate independence with maleness. Mays and Cochran (1987) list three solutions to this problem of cultural orientation:

1. Include family and friends in education and treatment efforts.
2. Create an atmosphere that invites questions from patients, to assist them in overcoming the tendency to feel ignorant or bothersome in patient education situations. Ask for questions, repeat important concepts to the patient, as well as to his/her significant others, in the most simple language possible.
3. Review basic AIDS information frequently, to check for accuracy and understanding.

Orlando Taylor (1987) has developed a list of verbal and non-verbal communication styles of working class Black Americans (see Table I). These language patterns have been contrasted with Anglo- Americans and middle class persons of other ethnic groups. The list is not exhaustive and Taylor reminds readers to allow for individual variations within both cultures and to avoid generalizations and stereotypes. An awareness of these

Table I.   Examples of Verbal and Nonverbal Communication Contrasts Among
            Some Black Americans and Some Anglo-Americans

Some Black Americans

• Hats and sunglasses may be considered by men as adornments much like jewelry, and may be worn indoors

• Touching another's hair is considered offensive

• Asking personal questions of a person met for the first time may be seen as improper and intrusive

• Use of direct questions is sometimes considered harassment (e.g., asking when something will be finished is like rushing that person to finish)

Some Anglo-Americans

• Hats and sunglasses are considered utilitarian by men; and as outerwear to be removed indoors

• Touching another's hair is a sign of affection

• Inquiring about jobs, family, and so forth of someone one has met for the first time is seen as friendly

• Use of direct questions for personal information is permissible

- The term "you people" is typically seen as pejorative and racist

- Listeners are expected to avert eyes to indicate respect and attention

- Talking "Black" by outsiders without authorization is an insult

- Showing emotions during conflict is acceptable, perceived as honesty, and viewed as the first step toward the the resolution of a problem

- The term "you people" is tolerated

- Listeners are expected to look at speaker directly to indicate respect and attention

- Borrowing of language forms from another group is permissible and encouraged

- Showing emotions during conflict is perceived as the beginning of a "fight," discordant, and an interference to conflict resolution

Source: Taylor, O.L. (1987). Cross-cultural communication: An essential dimension of effective education. Washington, DC: The American University.

differences in communication styles can assist health care professionals in identifying and correctly interpreting these behaviors.

Hispanic Americans

The Hispanic population, which currently numbers 19 million in the United States is the fastest growing segment of the American population (The National Coalition of Hispanic Health and Human Services Organizations [COSSMHO], 1988). Hispanic is a relatively new, generic term which refers to persons of Spanish origin or descent. In the 1985 Census, Hispanics were subdivided into five categories to include:

- Mexican or Mexican-Americans, or Chicano;
- Puerto Rican;
- Cuban or Cuban-American;
- Central or South American; and
- "Other" Spanish/Hispanic.

Of the 19 million Hispanics who live in the United States, 63% are Mexican-American, 12% are Puerto Rican, 5% Cuban, 10% Central and South American and 8% "other hispanic" (COSSMHO, 1988). It is important to remember that, like other cultural groups, Hispanics are a heterogeneous population despite the fact that they share some commonalties in language, heritage, religion and values. Not all Hispanics, however, use Spanish as their first language, and some do not speak Spanish at all. Religious affiliation and church-related activity is important in the Hispanic community and approximately 85% identify themselves as Catholic.

Hispanics account for 14 percent of all reported AIDS cases and for 20% of AIDS cases among women and 23% of pediatric cases of AIDS. The rates among Hispanics appear to be related to intravenous drug abuse as 43% of Hispanic AIDS patients have IVDA as a risk factor as compared to 14% of non-Hispanic whites (COSSMHO, 1988).

Cultural Factors that Influence Hispanic Health

Balance and harmony in the physical, emotional and social spheres is considered essential to well-being in the Hispanic culture (Maduro, 1983). Illness and disease are often attributed to an imbalance in these factors. In the absence of access to mainstream health care, the services of folk healers may be sought in an effort to achieve the balance and harmony essential to health.

Home remedies are also an important part of the Hispanic culture. They are often used to treat fatigue, headache, edema, and gastrointestinal disturbances. In addition, many Hispanics, particularly of Latin American origin, highly value the role of the pharmacist, routinely consult them and seriously consider their recommendations. Medications are often shared among family members and friends without prior consultation with a professional. Hispanics typically expect observable results in medical care, such that if an individual feels better after a few days of medication, then they may discontinue its use. Also, Hispanics may discontinue use after a few days because they have experienced no observable result, even though the medication was intended to be for long-term administration, for example, an anti-hypertensive drug (COSSMHO, 1988).

Hispanics traditionally have had a very broad definition of "family." Family consists not only of spouse, children, parents and siblings; but also includes grandparents, aunts, uncles, cousins, godparents and close family friends. During illness, family members are often brought along for medical visits, even when the patient is an adult. When visiting a sick relative at the hospital, the family may come as a group of five or more people. This familism over individualism emphasizes interdependence and cooperation over independence and competition (Falicov, 1982). Important decisions are made as a family, not by an individual him/herself, and family members expect to be involved in the care of their ill member.

Formal rules in the Hispanic culture dictate the nature of interpersonal behavior. For example, the young are expected to show respect for their elders, women for men, students for teachers, and employees for employers. Health care providers are accorded respect as authority figures on the basis of their education and healing function. However, Hispanics expect that health care providers will demonstrate reciprocal respect for them by addressing them formally as "Senor" or "Senora" and listening attentively to their needs and concerns. This formality of address, however, does not indicate a desire for aloofness or distance in the relationship. In actuality, Hispanics tend to emphasize personal rather than impersonal relationships with their health care providers.

Continuity of care is also important as Hispanics often prefer, sometimes vehemently, to have the same physician/nurse/therapist provide their care over time. A consequence of the respect afforded to health care providers by many Hispanic individuals is the hesitancy to ask questions, express doubts about the treatment provided or disagree with the health care professional. Many avoid admitting confusion regarding instructions or treatment regimen. In addition, there is a taboo regarding the expression of negative feelings directly. As a result, the individual may withhold information, be noncompliant or terminate medical care (COSSMHO, 1988).

Nonverbal communication in the Hispanic culture typically includes physical touching, especially hugging, avoidance of eye contact with authority figures (out of respect), physical proximity as opposed to distance during interpersonal interaction, and a more open expression of pain than other ethnic groups. In general, Hispanics tend to be particularly aware of and sensitive to non-verbal communication.

Implications for Health Care Providers

1. Since not all Hispanics speak Spanish, find out which language individuals prefer to use; do not assume that they will prefer Spanish.
2. Hispanics often do not differentiate between modern medical care and folk and home remedies. Therefore, it is usually not helpful to ask them if they use "folk medicine;" rather, ask what medicines or herbs they are currently using.
3. Respect and affirm the individual and family's effort at self-care, rather than denigrate their use of folk or home remedies. This sets a tone of cooperation rather than antagonism.
4. Utilize culturally sensitive pamphlets, posters and other health education materials. This may include the use of Hispanic individuals in photographs and bilingual materials.
5. Include the extended family and church in the treatment process, as important decisions are primarily made as a family system.
6. Be sensitive to interpersonal communication issues, both verbal and non-verbal.

AIDS AND SUBSTANCE ABUSERS

The relationship between AIDS and substance abuse goes well beyond the clear-cut association with intravenous drug abuse and needle-sharing behavior (National Research Council, 1989; National Institute on Alcohol Abuse and Alcoholism, 1988). It is now known that substance abuse is implicated in the transmission of HIV through several indirect routes as well. For example, many if not all, psychoactive substances act as disinhibitors of sexual behavior. The use of these substances tends to diminish one's inhibitions and judgment and thereby increase the likelihood of irresponsible and high risk behavior, especially in the sexual arena (National Association of State Alcohol and Drug Abuse Directors [NASADAD], 1987). In addition, it is not uncommon in the drug culture to exchange sexual favors for drugs in order to supply an addiction. As the number of sexual partners increases so does the risk of HIV transmission. Recent evidence suggests that several drugs, most notably alcohol and the nitrite inhalants actually suppress the immune system and thereby increase the risk of HIV infection (National Research Council, 1989; National Institute on Alcohol Abuse and Alcoholism, 1988).

Intravenous Drug Abusers

Intravenous drug abuse has recently been cited as the leading mode of HIV transmission in the United States today by the Presidential Commission on the Human Immunodeficiency Virus Epidemic (American Medical Association, 1988). Currently, the National Institute on Drug Abuse estimates that there are 1.2 million IV drug users in the United States. This figure is not limited to the use of heroin, which is the drug most commonly administered in this way, but also includes the injection of cocaine and some amphetamines, particularly methamphetamine or "crank."

Injection of contaminated blood is probably the single most efficient means of transmitting the AIDS virus. The injection ritual often involves injecting a small amount of the drug, then drawing blood back into the syringe and repeating the process. This is referred to as "playing" or "booting" in the drug subculture and is done to slowly build the drug effect. This ritual permits small amounts of blood to remain in the syringe which when used by another addict increases the likelihood of HIV transmission.

In the year ending January 1, 1989, 23.7% of all AIDS cases reported were IV drug abusers and in New York City an estimated 61% of IVDA were HIV positive. Among this group, women and men appear to be equally susceptible to HIV infection (National Research Council, 1989).

Cultural Aspects of the IVDA Population

The transmission of HIV infection within the intravenous drug abuse (IVDA) population is the result of the sharing of contaminated "works" or drug injection needles which is a routine and highly valued activity in the IVDA subculture. Needle sharing studies indicate that somewhere between 50 and 99% of IVDAs engage in this practice (Haverkos, 1988). Needle sharing serves many functions including decreased possibility of arrest as possession of drug paraphernalia is illegal in all fifty states. Sharing also decreases economic expense in purchasing needles and socially it binds IVDAs in temporary but often intense personal relationships. Frequency of injection and environment, for example "shooting galleries," appear to be the best predictors of IVDA induced HIV infection (American Medical Association, 1988).

In addition to needle-sharing, other practices associated with IVDA also increase the risk of HIV infection. IVDAs often combine sexual activity with drug use and exchange sexual services in order to obtain drugs. For this reason, the transmission of HIV has spread to include the sexual partners of the IVDAs (primarily heterosexual women) and perinatal transmission to newborns born to IVDAs or their infected partners (American Public Health Association, 1989).

Other Considerations

In addition to the specific characteristics of the IVDA culture, the issues relevant to the drug culture in general are relevant in any consideration of AIDS.

Stigmatization has long been a barrier for alcohol and drug abusers seeking treatment. An alcohol or other drug abuser with AIDS is doubly stigmatized and is likely to be hostile, angry and uncooperative.

Denial is a major feature of chemical dependence. This denial is substantially different from the normal denial an individual experiences as part of the grief reaction associated with a terminal diagnosis. It is important to be able to distinguish between the denial associated with the diagnosis of AIDS, which is a normal defense mechanism and the denial associated with chemical dependence which is pathological and counterproductive. Often it may be that the individual with AIDS is not dealing with his/her own addiction but that of a partner or lover. Denial may be just as strong in this situation and must be addressed directly.

In addition, addicted clients/patients may be manipulative, pseudo-cooperative, non-cooperative or actively resistant to any intervention. This is another characteristic of the disease of chemical dependence. It is not unusual for such individuals to exaggerate pain symptoms, and complain about and/or change physicians in order to obtain large amounts of psychoactive pain medications.

Depression is another common feature of chemical dependence. Addicted individuals are at greater risk of committing suicide, and the normal grief reactions associated with a terminal illness are often exaggerated by chemical use.

According to the National Institute of Alcohol and Alcohol Abuse (1988), there is a clear underestimation of the amount of alcohol and other drug use among persons with AIDS and individuals infected with HIV. Alcohol and drug problems in AIDS patients often are unrecognized and untreated, possibly because, as health care providers, we are often reluctant to obtain drug and alcohol use histories.

When some health care providers do recognize an alcohol and/or a drug problem in an AIDS patient, the sense of hopelessness still associated with the diagnosis of AIDS may preclude treatment of the chemical dependence. This perspective overlooks the possibility that many of the medical and psychological problems of a person with AIDS may be associated with chemical dependence and may be alleviated through substance abuse treatment. This can have a profound effect on the quality of life for the individual and his/her friends and family.

The withdrawal syndrome from psychoactive substances varies depending on the specific drug. Symptoms may range from mild, flu-like discomfort to delirium tremens and profound depression. When an individual is admitted to a hospital for AIDS-related medical problems, withdrawal may ensue if the patient is also addicted to alcohol or other drugs. This can pose significant medical and psychological hazards and must be treated seriously.

Implications for Health Care Providers

1. The use of alcohol and other drugs further decreases the effectiveness of the immune system and therefore support for abstinence from psychoactive substances is essential in the treatment of AIDS. Participation in the Alcoholics Anonymous and Narcotics Anonymous support groups should be encouraged.
2. Confront the denial around AIDS gently with caring concern, but confront the denial surrounding chemical dependence and substance abuse with firmness and "tough love." Be sensitive to the fact that accepting a diagnosis of AIDS and acknowledging a substance abuse problem simultaneously may be too much stress for an individual to handle and act accordingly.
3. Health care providers must be alert to the signs of impending suicide as this population is at increased risk.
4. Health care providers must become more aware of the dynamics of chemical dependence and the behavioral and psychological manifestations of the disease.
5. Drug treatment programs need to incorporate not only AIDS education, but also support for behavior change, for example, role playing, skill building and support groups.
6. AIDS treatment programs need to incorporate chemical dependence education for staff, patients and their families.
7. In addition, the needs of sexual partners and children must be con-

sidered. AIDS must be addressed as a family issue where alcohol and other drug abuse is involved. In these family units prevention education, risk reduction and family support strategies are essential.

AIDS AND THE GAY/HOMOSEXUAL COMMUNITY

According to the National Research Council (1989), HIV prevalence rates among homosexual and bisexual males ranges from 20 to 50 percent across 23 cities in 16 states. With these rates the health care system will continue to treat Gay males with AIDS for many years to come. Transmission of HIV among this group is primarily through unprotected receptive anal intercourse. Increased risk of HIV infection is associated with having a large number of sexual partners; the use of bath houses for sexual contacts; current infection with other sexually transmitted diseases and the use of inhaled nitrites (National Research Council, 1989).

Cultural Aspects of the Gay Community

Research indicates that among gay and bisexual males the rates of multiple sex partners are much greater than in the heterosexual population (National Research Council, 1989). In a study conducted in San Francisco, 26.8% of gay men reported having 10 or more partners in the preceding six months while the number of heterosexual males reporting the same number of sexual partners was 2.8% (Winklestein et al., 1987). In recent national studies, significant declines in the average number of sexual partners of gay men have been noted (National Research Council, 1989). Studies have also shown a dramatic decline in HIV transmission among gay and bisexual men, notably due to increased educational efforts targeted towards enhancing safer sex practices (Institute of Medicine, 1988).

In heterosexual society, a person's development is often evaluated based on a predetermined pattern built around the nuclear family. The nuclear family model is not appropriate in the Gay community. A more workable alternative has been the development of gay friendship networks and support groups. These networks can be extensive and are not based solely on sexual relationships. They serve multiple purposes, including fulfilling needs for safety and security, affiliation and love.

Stereotypes of gay males tend to include such descriptors as "effeminate," "promiscuous," and "flamboyant," but the range of personalities in the gay community is no different than in the heterosexual community. Gays come from every culture, religion, ethnic group and occupational status. Gay relationships do not follow typical male-female roles as in heterosexual society, so it is inappropriate to assume that one person in the relationship "plays" the role of husband, and the other the role of "wife."

A diagnosis of HIV or AIDS may force an individual to openly confront his homosexuality for the first time publicly. It may be the first time that family members, friends and co-workers become aware of the individual as a gay person. This "coming out" process can magnify an already stressful situation, and health care providers need to be sensitive to such concerns.

Implications for Health Care Providers

1. If you are unfamiliar with the gay culture, admit this to the patient. An interest in another person's lifestyle and a willingness to learn can foster a positive therapeutic relationship.
2. Avoid overgeneralizations and stereotypes and treat each individual as unique. Moral debates regarding sexual behaviors and a condescending attitude have no place in the health care arena.
3. Re-define your concept of family to include gay lovers and friends and encourage their visitation and participation in the care of the patient.
4. Use appropriate sexual terminology and avoid sexual comments and innuendo.

CONCLUSION

Although these three sub-populations have been discussed as if they were separate and distinct, it must be noted that persons with AIDS may belong to more than one of these cultural groups. It is not uncommon for a Black male with AIDS to also be an IV drug user, or for a Gay male with AIDS to be an alcoholic. A variety of such combinations is possible and so it becomes imperative that health care providers learn as much as possible about these cultural groups and include these considerations in the evaluation and treatment of persons with AIDS.

Individuals who practice high-risk behaviors for HIV infection often have life-styles quite different from the health care providers who care for them. Only by becoming more knowledgeable, sensitive and accepting of alternative life-styles and cultural issues can professionals provide compassionate and effective assistance.

ESSAY QUESTIONS

1. *Describe how and why cultural considerations are relevant in the treatment of persons with AIDS.*
2. *Compare and contrast the health-related beliefs of Black Americans and Hispanic Americans and describe how these beliefs can affect patient-provider interactions.*
3. *Discuss the ways in which AIDS and alcohol/drug abuse are directly and indirectly related.*
4. *Describe the ways in which the Gay/homosexual culture is different from the mainstream heterosexual society and how this impacts the treatment of persons with AIDS.*

REFERENCES

American Medical Association. (1988, September). Intravenous drug abuse and AIDS. *The Reporter*. Chicago: AMA.

American Public Health Association. (1989, January). *Illicit Drug Use and HIV Infection*. Washington, DC: APHA.

Back, Gloria, G. (1985). *Are You Still My Mother? Are You Still My Family?* New York: Warner Books.

Berzon, Betty, ed. (1979). *Positively Gay*. Los Angeles, CA: Mediamix Associates.

Cope, N.R. and Hall, H.R. (1985). The health status of Black women in the U.S.: Implications for health psychology and behavioral medicine. *SAGE: A Scholarly Journal on Black Women*, 2 (2), 20-24.

COSSMHO National Coalition of Hispanic Health and Human Services Organization. (1988). *Delivering Preventive Health Care to Hispanics: A Manual for Providers*. Washington, DC: COSSMHO.

Dixon, V.J., King, L.M., and Nobles, W.W. (1976). *African Philosophy: Assumptions and Paradigms for Research on Black Persons*. Los Angeles: Fanon Center Publication.

Falicov, C.J. (1982). Mexican families. In M. McGoldrick; J.K. Pearce; and J. Giordano (Eds.), *Ethnicity and Family Therapy*, 134-163. New York: Guilford Press.

Foster, B. (1971). Toward a definition of Black referents. In V.J. Dixon & Foster, B.G. (Eds.) *Beyond Black or White: An Alternate America*. (pp.9-22). Boston, MA: Little, Brown and Company.

Haverkos, H.W. (1988). Overview: HIV infection among intravenous drug abusers in the United States and Europe. In R.J. Battjes and R.W. Pickens (Eds.), *Needle Sharing among Intravenous Drug Abusers: National and International Perspectives*. Washington DC: Government Printing Office.

Institute of Medicine. (1988). Confronting AIDS: update 1988. Washington, D.C.: National Academy Press.

Leads from the MMWR. (1989). Distribution of AIDS cases by racial/ethnic group and exposure category, United States, June 1, 1981-July 4, 1988. *Journal of the American Medical Association*, 261(2), 201-205.

Maduro, R. (1983). Curanderismo and Latino views of disease and curing. *The Western Journal of Medicine*. 139,(6): 868-874.

Mays, V.M. and Cochran, S.D. (1987). Acquired immunodeficiency syndrome and black americans: Special psychosocial issues. *Public Health Reports*, 102(2), 224-31.

National Association of State Alcohol and Drug Abuse Directors, NASADAD (1987). Testimony of Joseph E. Mills III, Director, Division of Addiction Services, State of Indiana before the Presidential Commission on the Human Immunodeficiency Virus Epidemic, December 18, 1987.

National Institute on Alcohol and Alcohol Abuse. (1988). *Acquired Immune Deficiency Syndrome and Chemical Dependency*. Washington, DC: Government Printing Office.

National Institute on Drug Abuse. (1987). *Drug Abuse and Drug Abuse Research*. Washington, DC: Government Printing Office.

National Research Council. (1989). *AIDS: Sexual Behavior and Intravenous Drug Use*. Washington, DC: National Academy Press.

Snow, L.F. (1983). Traditional health beliefs and practices among lower class black americans. *Western Journal of Medicine*, 139(6), 820-8.

Snow, L.F. (1974). Folk medical beliefs and their implications for care of patients. *Annals of Internal Medicine*, 81, 82-96.

Taylor, O.L. (1987). *Cross-Cultural Communication: An Essential Dimension of Effective Education*. Washington, DC: The American University.

United States Department of Health and Human Services. (1985). *Report of the Secretary's Task Force on Black and Minority Health. Volume II: Crosscutting Issues in Minority Health*. Washington, DC: Government Printing Office.

United States Department of Health and Human Services. (1986). *Report of the Secretary's Task Force on Black and Minority Health. Volume VIII: Hispanic Health Survey*. Washington, DC: Government Printing Office.

Winkelstein, W., Jr., Samuel, M., Padian, N.S., and Wiley, J.A. (1987). Selected sexual practices of San Francisco hetero-sexual men and risk of infection by the human immunodeficiency virus. *Journal of the American Medical Association*, 257: 1470-1471.

Wright, R. (1984). *African Philosophy: An Introduction*. (pp. 50-3). Lanham, MD: University Press of America.

AIDS:
The Spiritual Challenge

Holly L. Presti, OTR

SUMMARY. Three primary spiritual aspects of HIV and AIDS are guilt, perceived experiential losses, and the search for meaning. The founding theoretical principles of occupational therapy, including moral treatment, are combined with spiritual components in this paper. The meaning of occupation and activities are discussed. Emphasis is placed on hope and its effect on restoration of health in relation to the maximum functioning of the immune system. Occupational therapy combined with reaching spiritual well-being, which contributes to the quality of life, are seen as methods by which optimum health is achieved.

INTRODUCTION

The onset of the AIDS epidemic has changed man's perception of illness. It has caused people to probe deeper into the soul than any other illness in modern history. Whether a child, adult, or caregiver, the impact of AIDS will be experienced in a spiritual dimension. In dealing with AIDS one is forced to deal with life and death issues. For many, this becomes a spiritual experience: it transcends what is trivial and grasps at the eternal and that which lies beyond. Whether AIDS is known to us as a disease "somebody else gets" or a disease that killed a best friend, or we

---

Holly L. Presti is Senior Occupational Therapist at the Robert Wood Johnson University Hospital, New Brunswick, NJ.
The author wishes to gratefully acknowledge the support and assistance of Cindy Jarvis, Jack Guarneri, Alison Alaimo, and David Presti.
The author acknowledges that AIDS is the final stage of HIV infection. AIDS is used throughout this article for consistency, and does not imply that only people with AIDS encounter spiritual dilemmas, but that people with HIV or other conditions encounter spiritual dilemmas as well.

are afflicted with it ourselves, it causes all whom it affects to board a spiritual journey.

Spiritual Defined

In *AIDS, The Spiritual Dilemma*, John Fortunato (1987) states that *spiritual* "is such a loaded term. People use it to refer to anything from the phantasmagoric mystical experiences of hermits in caves to evangelical — pentecostal — charismatic fervor" (Fortunato, 1987, p. 7). In this article, neither of these definitions is intended when the word is used; rather, *spiritual* is meant to signify something both rational and profoundly *felt* by an individual who has had to confront AIDS. This article is an attempt to look beyond the medical, psychosocial, cultural, and pastoral facts and provide a glimpse of the reality of AIDS in perhaps its broadest context — the spiritual realm. This includes man's need for belonging, transcendence, sense of meaning and purpose, and need for creativity (Bowers, 1987). It includes all the spiritual aspects experienced by the person with AIDS, the family, the friends, and the health care worker.

All men and women are spiritual beings (Vaillot, 1970; Jourard, S.M., 1964). They have a need for grounding, some deep sense of belonging (Powell, 1978). Fortunato describes it as follows:

> . . . the journey of the soul — not to religion itself but to the drive in humankind that gives rise to religion in the first place . . . that aura around all of our lives that gives what we do meaning, the human striving toward meaning, the search for a sense of belonging. (Fortunato, 1987, p. 7-8)

Many psychologists believe that there is within each person a drive to self-actualize his or her potentialities (Johnson, 1981). Does anyone ever achieve this state? Is it not precisely the very striving for this peak that keeps one going? Perhaps it is this journey that is the very path men and women take when they seek meaning in life (Powell, 1978).

This article seeks to address three primary spiritual issues: guilt, perceived experiential losses, and the search for meaning. Guilt is at the forefront of many personal experiences with AIDS. It is consistently identified by professionals working with people with AIDS as a primary spiritual issue. The perceived losses are also a spiritual issue of major importance. Rejection, its resulting isolation, alienation, and physical deterioration lead to a profound sense of loss. The next step in the natural progression is looking for the hope, the purpose, the meaning in all of this.

One often postpones a serious examination of the meaning of life or such related spiritual issues until the onset of a severe illness (Snow, 1987). When life and death are personally faced, one is forced to make spiritual decisions; to do some spiritual problem-solving. When faced with serious illness, people need to "make sense of their circumstances and find meaning in the events of one's day, one's relationships, one's life . . ." (Simsen, 1988, p. 31).

In *AIDS, The Ultimate Challenge*, Kubler-Ross (1987) gives an account of dealing with the spiritual aspects from the point of view of a caregiver who is describing a spiritual experience. While the caregiver and other volunteers were in the room of a dying person, touching and holding hands, the caregiver noticed she was

> . . . sitting in the midst of what life is really supposed to be all about . . . loving, caring, supporting, sharing . . . involved on such a level of unconditional love and support . . . coming in contact with that space inside of us that is pure unconditional love. . . . It's what life is all about. (Kubler-Ross, 1987, p. 277)

AIDS causes caregivers, families, friends, and neighbors to examine the spiritual struggle and the spiritual response in their broadest, most inclusive definitions.

REVIEW OF THE LITERATURE

In reviewing the literature and interviewing pastors, church members, and others providing spiritual care to persons affected by AIDS, numerous common spiritual issues can be identified. They include dealing with the stigma surrounding AIDS (Shelp, 1986; Marshall & Nieckarz, 1988; Fortunato, 1987), rejection (Marshall, 1987; Gaze, 1987; Kubler-Ross, 1987), and alienation, isolation and loneliness (Marshall, 1987; Hamilton, 1988; Amos, 1988; D'Aloisio, 1989). Other issues are the withdrawal of the self or of others (Kubler-Ross, 1987) and the resulting lack of support systems (Shelp, 1986). People affected by a terminal illness such as AIDS often must deal with anger (Ferszt & Taylor, 1988), denial, and a profound sense of loss of control (Bowers, 1987). They may experience guilt (Kubler-Ross, 1987; Fortunato, 1987), a sense of shame, or a lack of self worth (Snow, 1987). They may glimpse a sense of their own finitude for the first time in their lives (Fortunato, 1987).

In contrast, the person affected by AIDS may experience a renewed sense of peace through reconciled relationships (Shelp, 1986). He or she may experience new spiritual growth (Shelp, 1986; Scott, 1988; Weinstein, 1989) or, more specifically, an inner drive to search for explanation, fulfillment, meaning (Fortunato, 1987; Simsen, 1988; Pizzi, 1988).

Occupational therapy plays an important role in addressing these spiritual issues and in facilitating an adaptive response. These issues bring a reminder of the sense of the human condition – of what it is to be human and finite. Exploration of these issues brings an understanding of man's communion or lack of communion with his world and his God. AIDS may involve dealing with many cultural, medical, and psychosocial issues, to name only a few. The spiritual aspects, however, are those that reach to a person's core.

PRIMARY SPIRITUAL ISSUES

Guilt

The guilt associated with AIDS is a major spiritual issue for many people. The origins of guilt are complex. Often they are related to parental standards, cultural mores, and religious upbringing (Haburchak et al., 1989). It may be the guilt of a chosen lifestyle – possibly that which caused infection. It may include guilt of infecting others. It may be the guilt of being homosexual, bisexual, a drug user, or withheld communications such as never having disclosed one's sexuality or use of illegal substances to family members and friends. Disclosing one's lifestyle combined with disclosure of having a chronic and often fatal illness can exacerbate guilt.

Guilt may stem from a feeling of being punished by God. The person may believe that, due to certain behaviors, a diagnosis of HIV infection was deserved. While some people of faith may encourage this thought by their moralistic views, AIDS is no indication of God's view of behavior. "God did not send AIDS, chicken pox, or small pox on any particular person or group of people. If it rains, some people will get wet. It's as simple as that" (Shelp, 1986, p. 59).

For the homosexual, the ability to cope with AIDS and the consequent guilt often appears to depend on his sense of ease or uncertainty with his sexuality. Often a man who has reconciled his sexuality and his spirituality prior to his HIV positive diagnosis is further developed, spiritually, and is therefore able to deal with the issues of dying more effectively (D. Davis, personal communication, August 23, 1989; D. Wall, personal communication, September 1, 1989). Yet, one chaplain has consistently found in her work that even patients who were told they were forgiven by friends and families, and reported having a close relationship with God and an active prayer life, were unable to get beyond their own feelings of guilt and forgive themselves (A. Bauerband, personal communication, September 14, 1989).

The person with AIDS who experiences guilt often has an extremely low sense of self worth and may see him or herself as worthless. The perception of self may be so dysfunctional that it may interfere with the individual's social and occupational functioning.

For the parents of a child with AIDS, feelings of guilt may abound. They may feel responsible for the contaminated blood supply with which the child was transfused. They may feel they were not careful enough in their own behaviors, which led to infection in their young. And, their guilt may also affect their social and occupational functioning.

Loss

The person with AIDS experiences a profound sense of loss. Losses may include the loss of physical abilities, mental functioning, or physical beauty. The loss of a particular and familiar role may occur as one's role in the family, in social relationships, and in the workplace change with the progression of the illness (Pizzi, 1989). While some may experience loss of role at work, many experience loss of job, and with that, loss of insurance and the security of knowing that financial needs will be met. Often there is loss of housing. The sense of privacy is often lost, especially with the manifestation of Kaposi's sarcoma or weight loss, repeated hospitalizations, and possible disclosure of one's once private lifestyle, which may be "different" from the norm.

One may experience the loss of support systems. The person with AIDS may experience multiple deaths of friends and loved ones. One man, ill with numerous opportunistic infections actually welcomed the progression of his illness, which made him bedridden, because attending so many funerals was too devastating and intense to bear (Kubler-Ross, 1987). Another loss of friends may occur because of friends' fear of infection, or friends' lack of understanding of the disease or of a lifestyle now exposed, or because of an inability to face being reminded of one's own mortality (Shelp, 1986).

Loss may occur in the lack of family support. Alienation by a family may occur due to its devastation upon learning of a son's drug use, sexual preference, or inability to cope with an AIDS diagnosis. They withdraw love and contact when needed most. As one nurse reports, in most of the cases she has seen involving homosexuals, AIDS permanently divided the family (Garrett, 1988). Lack of family support may also occur no matter how the disease was contracted. Families do not know what to say to the aunts and uncles when a baby with HIV infection is repeatedly hospitalized. Rather than risk rejection and ultimate isolation, many people will simply inform others that they have cancer, or make reference to an unnamed serious illness (Garrett, 1988).

Coupled with the losses of support of friends and family is the loss of community, often the faith community. Jean Smith, an Episcopal minister, perceives alienation and isolation caused by the loss of support systems as the major spiritual issue facing the people who are influenced directly by AIDS (J. Smith, personal communication, September 13, 1989). Although she does not doubt her church members' willingness to respond to the needs of someone with AIDS, she admits to their hesitancy. She acknowledges their difficulty in dealing with personal biases and lack of knowledge about the illness, stressing the need for more education. Other pastors or rabbis may be less welcoming, and rejection may be preached from the pulpit. This may include incorrect assumptions relating behavior and diagnosis (Tapia, 1988). Tapia notes in his pamphlet, *The AIDS Crisis*, that "proposals by Christians to quarantine those with AIDS . . . is a deplorable attitude by the very ones who could provide the greatest hope and comfort for the sufferers" (Tapia, 1988, p. 14). Fortunately, the view of AIDS as God's judgment is nearly uniformly rejected by people directly or indirectly affected by the disease (Shelp, 1986).

The numerous accounts of church leaders, rejecting and condemning people with AIDS from the pulpit or on television unfortunately persist (Tapia, 1988; Shelp, 1986). It is then that people with AIDS may lose all hope — for when the house of God rejects them, they sense that God himself has rejected them. It is perceived as an ultimate sense of alienation and abandonment. Yet, perhaps, at this point one may be propelled into action or into a deeper search for meaning.

One mother, within the weeks that followed her son's death from AIDS, committed herself to work to help find a cure for AIDS. She talked with people, shared information regarding the latest medical advances, and educated people about prevention. So much of what she attempted, however, was met by obstacles. In her grief and loss of strength, she turned to personal prayer. Additionally, she established a day of prayer with the clergy association in her locale. This was met with tremendous support. It provided hope, which relieved some of her despair (M. Van Dagens, personal communication, October 5, 1989).

Shelp (1986) states in *AIDS, Personal Stories in Pastoral Perspective*, that because of the many negative responses of religious groups to AIDS, people with AIDS often "take refuge directly in God, rather than in the institutions and the people who claim to represent God" (Shelp, 1986, p. 184).

Search for Meaning

Losing ten close friends in a year to AIDS, seeing one's own body wither away from the disease, or seeing every other bed in the hospital in which one works fill up with people with AIDS, causes one to look for meaning, purpose, and hope in everyday living. The person with AIDS often feels hopeless, yet at times it is through this very lack of hope that one finds the compassion and support of others. Ultimately, most spiritual quests, while differing perhaps in rituals, religious language, or traditional customs, have the same basic spiritual questions and needs (Ferszt & Taylor, 1988). These usually focus on the search for hope (Bowers, 1987; Sodestrom and Martinson, 1987).

The search for meaning and hope may begin with questioning the purpose for the disease itself. Some suggest it is to allow humans to show unconditional love to one another; it has given a cause for compassion (Kubler-Ross, 1987; Shelp, 1987). Still others may wonder if AIDS is the result of bad parenting or deviant behavior (Garrett, 1988).

Linda Gutterman, an occupational therapist working with people with AIDS states that ". . . there's a lot about healing that doesn't always mean someone gets better physically. There has to be a spiritual component — a part that makes the client positive about his situation despite the negativeness of it" (D'Aloisio, 1989, p. 17). A counseling coordinator for the Shanti project, which provides the emotional support services for AIDS patients at San Francisco General Hospital, states, "to have someone just sit there and listen, and not try to fix it can be so healing" (McCaffrey, 1987, p. 26).

In an occupational therapist's study of people living with AIDS and people at risk, or with AIDS-Related Complex (ARC), 33% of the respondents report having been able to live more fully and appreciate life more. An additional 13% of the group studied felt they were brought "closer to God" because of AIDS. When asked who or what helped most in dealing with death and dying with AIDS, 47% reported religion, spirituality, priest, church, or prayer (Weinstein, 1989). AIDS has brought people beyond the contemplation of the temporal and into the eternal.

Positive aspects of the search for meaning may include reconciliation with friends, family members, or God. One man confesses that if he had never contracted AIDS, he never would have become closer to God or healed broken relationships or heard his mother tell him she loved him.

Other stories include numerous accounts of being flooded with the kindness and compassion of others, being able to live life more fully — to notice everything in creation with a renewed, "elevated level of conscious awareness" (Shelp, 1986, p. 91). AIDS enabled one patient to find God and become a person able to separate the important from the trivial (Weinstein, 1989). Another states that AIDS "is the best thing that has ever happened to me. It enabled me to break my addiction to methamphetamines" (Shelp, 1986, p. 31). Others say they have found meaning in learning how vulnerable life is, how to sympathize with minorities, how to love purely (Shelp, 1986).

The search for meaning may involve organized religious groups, but in many cases, one's spiritual search for meaning is private and individual. Still, either as caregivers, friends, family members, or members of the health care team, individuals can assist in channeling hope into the healing process by encouraging the AIDS-afflicted person to seek answers with spiritual guidance.

In the context of meaning, effective treatment can take place. As Meyer (cited in Engelbardt, 1983) stated, even activities which may appear trivial can endow time with meaning. Meaningful activity can allow patients to retake possession of their skills and capacity for productive use of time (Engelhardt, 1983). Occupational therapy is based on this premise.

THE SCOPE OF OCCUPATIONAL THERAPY

The Meaning of Occupation

The needs of a person who has AIDS are great. There are many physical needs which may include the need for assistance with daily tasks such as eating, bathing, and dressing. Needs expand beyond that and may include the need for financial help or housing. The list of needs is extensive. There are many social and psychological needs as well. Occupational therapists have traditionally looked at the whole person. Therapists pride themselves on attempting to include all aspects of daily living skills in treatment whose aim espouses that all needs should be met, all dysfunctional limbs should work again, all appropriate behaviors should be exhibited, and all activities of daily living should be performed independently.

Occupational therapists, therefore, need to more closely examine the "purposeful activity" engaged in by the recipients of treatment. The activity and their performance in a purposeful task should assist in giving clients a reason to get up each day. A crucial principle for therapists to acknowledge and incorporate into therapy is the fact that what a patient initially finds meaningful will be generated out of practical interest. This, subsequently, provides the foundation for an effective reconstruction of meaning (Sharrott, 1983).

In addition, therapy should "foster the externalizations of self beyond those predicated on disability" (Sharrott, 1983, p. 232). Occupational therapy must transcend the immediate experiences of the clinic or the rehabilitation process. Pursuit in therapy incorporating interests, valued goals, or personal or career objectives provides substance for the transition to functioning in society along an adaptive continuum (Sharrott, 1983).

It should also be noted, as cited by Nelson (1988), that all activities are not equal in terms of their puposefulness. Nelson takes the position that a person's individual developmental structure influences the degree of purpose a specific activity may have for certain individuals. The role of occupational therapy is to provide the client with an appropriate activity. For example, Yerxa explained authentic occupational therapy by the following:

> Through the use of media the client is involved intellectually and emotionally in discovering what is purposeful to him. He is also involved in relation to objects, actions and persons. Through these relationships he is helped to come to grips with his particular reality including his disability, his emotional reactions, his will and his potential. (Yerxa, 1984, p. 170-171)

Yerxa emphasizes the "will" which correlates with drive, inner need, or sense of purpose. Occupational therapy treatment rests on these principles.

Occupational Therapy and Immune Competency

If all the physical, psychological, and social needs are met, and there is still no hope for living each day, the treatment is incomplete. There needs to exist more than only an absence of illness. There must be a balance of systems, which not only protect from illness (one's immune system) but also lead to a healthy, fully functional, adaptive life.

People with AIDS are immunosuppressed. Their T-helper cells are being attacked. Simply stated, there are fewer T-cells. Additionally, the added stresses and prolonged illness or depression further suppresses T-cell competency, conclude Schleifer et al., and Stein (as cited in Farber, 1989).

Pearsall (cited in Farber, 1989) said that "superimmunity is the capacity to think and feel in ways that can protect us from disease, heal us when we are sick, and help us attain new levels of wellness . . . far beyond the mere absence of symptoms" (p. 639).

Recently, Farber (1989) examined the premises on which occupational therapy operates regarding the immunosuppressed person with AIDS. "Occupational therapists must examine whether positive, supportive attitudes influence patients in a manner that improves immune competency," suggests Farber (1989, p. 639). She goes on to state that

> We as occupational therapists, because of the nature of our holistic interaction with patients, are in a perfect position to foster the development of enhanced immunity. We can encourage patients to establish positive attitudes (empowerment) and reduce helplessness and hopelessness. This action might improve the patient's immune function. (Farber, 1989, p. 639)

Borysenko, (cited in Farber, 1989) found that emotional well-being can enhance immune function. Likewise, Cousins (1979; 1989) maintained that having hope and expectations affects the autonomic nervous system and body biochemistry. He cites the powerful effect of placebos as well. He states that in studies of AIDS patients who have lived far beyond initial diagnosis, there is documented increased activity of a wide range of immune cells other than those directly attacked by HIV. Other tests indicate actual enhancement of the T-cells and correlations between adaptive emotional attitudes (saying no to doom) and better immune measures (including increased numbers of helper T-cells) (Cousins, 1989).

Therefore, it appears that concern and compassionate holistic treatment for persons with AIDS may bring about biochemical changes in the body which result in the production of more T-helper cells. More T-helper cells may increase a person's immunologic response to illness as well as add to a person's quality of life by enabling him or her to "live more fully," with a more complete sense of well-being, health, healing.

While realizing that AIDS cannot be made extinct by an "enhanced immunity" alone, these claims provide evidence for the power that is available in coping with any life situation. One cannot help but apply it to even the spiritual realm with relation to AIDS.

Occupational Therapy: Facilitator of Hope

As previously discussed, persons affected by AIDS have spiritual needs. Often these needs surround the search for meaning, purpose, and hope. There are many ways in which occupational therapists provide hope. One method may involve improving a person's physical and psychological functioning. Often, with greater independence in daily tasks, one experiences improved self-esteem and increased motivation (Hopkins, 1978). William Rush Dunton, Jr. stated in 1919 that one of the basic founding premises upon which occupational therapy was developed was that "sick minds, sick bodies, sick souls may be healed through occupation" (Hopkins, 1978, p. 11).

Occupational therapy can provide hope by increasing a person's capacity to deal with and adapt to illness. As Adolf Meyer indicated in the early 1900s, "conflicts in functioning occur through poor adaptation. Occupation may influence and enhance human adaptiveness" (Hopkins, 1978, p. 6). The person with AIDS may lose vital visual or cognitive skills, yet adapt to these losses by the use of compensatory strategies or other adaptive methods. The person who has lost physical endurance may be able to continue to function by employing energy conservation and work simplification techniques as taught by an occupational therapist. This person may benefit from instruction in time management principles and the appropriate balance of work and rest. Likewise, the pleasure of achievement, a real pleasure in the use of one's hands and muscles, and a happy appreciation of time are the incentives that have been used since the founding of occupational therapy (Meyer, 1922).

Occupational therapy's theoretical framework is inherently hopeful. It focuses on function, not on dysfunction. This relates to the philosophy, espoused by Cousins (1989), that focus must be on the possibilities of life instead of on the limitations. By increasing a person's awareness of strengths and skills that are intact, one can more effectively move toward optimum health. There is reassurance and encouragement when emphasis is placed on the positive. Ayres captures the power of hope in her emphasis on using the inner needs of a person as the method by which activities are chosen and therapeutically directed (Ayres, 1972).

Likewise, occupational therapy had its beginning in moral treatment which, in part, proposed that all patients be treated with dignity, respect, and kindness. Bing (1981) stated that

> The Quakers brought moral treatment to the United States as part of their intellectual and religious luggage. . . . During the last quarter of the nineteenth century moral treatment disappeared. It reemerged in the early decades of the twentieth century as Occupational Therapy. (Bing, 1981, p. 499)

Its purpose was to "create an atmosphere in which natural restorative elements could assert themselves" (Peloquin, 1989, p. 538). In most cases, it included manual labor, establishment of regular habits of self control, diversion of the mind from morbid thoughts, and attendance at *religious worship* (Peloquin, 1989). While the spiritual components of worship will not be examined here, it is to be acknowledged that worship focuses on what is beyond oneself and on a greater power. Worship embodies hope. The Occupational therapist can foster hope.

Occupational Therapy: A Resource

An important role of occupational therapists is to facilitate optimum functioning and adaptation to the environment. Adapting to the community may be especially difficult for the person with AIDS who lacks the necessary support systems or who may be rejected by organizations or institutions traditionally invoked for support. An occupational therapist knowledgeable about appropriate community resources can offer a wealth of hope for a person living with AIDS. If a person with AIDS is seeking concrete medical hope, perhaps his or her therapist could refer the client to a drug testing clinic or a doctor who specializes in experimental treatments for persons with AIDS. A patient may require extensive counseling beyond the expertise of an occupational therapist. This may lead to a referral to a psychiatrist, psychologist, social worker, or clergy. An occupational therapist cannot meet every need of the client. Clients are served best when a therapist realizes he or she is unable to meet every need and additional assistance is obtained.

The sources an occupational therapist may utilize in assisting a person with AIDS who is struggling with spiritual matters are the national, state and local organizations specifically designed to serve people with AIDS. Organizations are located throughout the country. They may offer a wide variety of services including such things as medical care, support groups, or a listing of trained clergy who are especially sensitive to the needs of people with AIDS. Another source is the organized church or synagogue. Churches and temples are beginning to respond more positively to the issues surrounding AIDS.

Many churches now have AIDS task forces or AIDS resource committees. They are coordinating educational forums and lecture series as part of the adult education program. They are addressing such issues as the medical aspects, the local statistics and needs, the congregation's involvement in assisting with homes for people with AIDS, the local hospital's response, and the raising of awareness of AIDS in the rest of the church at large and in the local community. Ministers and rabbis are speaking about AIDS with statements of compassion, appropriately grouping AIDS with other diseases, struggles, and matters which need prayer. Networks of volunteers are set up to visit people with AIDS, cook for them, take them to their doctors, clean their homes. One church ministered so warmly to a person with AIDS that after he died his friends, and their friends, attended the church regularly, further strengthening an AIDS support network (A. Bauerband, personal communication, September 14, 1989).

Churches and synagogues are supporting the community organizations serving people with AIDS. Some have linked with the pediatric AIDS programs to go to hospitals, where they visit, hold, and play with children who have AIDS. One church houses the office for the state-wide organization serving people with AIDS. Still another has an AIDS booktable with knowledgeable volunteers at its "coffee hour" on Sunday mornings. Educational programs within congregations have led to greater involvement by members in local AIDS organizations, dispelling the myths about AIDS and increasing openness and acceptance of people with various lifestyles.

Because the effects of AIDS are so broad, many varying disciplines and community resources are necessary in order to serve people with AIDS. Activity, involving mind and body, creativity, and socialization are valuable. Counseling as provided by mental health professionals or trained volunteers may be very effective. Advanced experimental treatments and new drugs may provide improved functioning and prolong life. Enhanced involvement in the faith community or in personal study may provide new inspiration. Yet all of these things may still not answer the inner yearning for meaning and purpose in life for people with AIDS. However, they may, collectively, lead the way to a spiritual understanding and sense of purpose that is so desperately sought by one who is dealing with his or her own finitude.

CONCLUSION

While this article cannot deal with the enormity of the spiritual issues and aspects of AIDS, it has hopefully given a sense of the depth of the spiritual challenge facing anyone affected by AIDS. When seeking to find what is spiritual or searching for a sense of closeness to a greater power, one may look to a synagogue, church, or go from one technique to another expert, or from one discipline to a silent retreat. The point is, however, that in a spiritual search, people look for basically the same things. They are seeking hope, meaning, purpose: a sense that their life matters. We would do well to remember the story of Jesus eating with sinners, prostitutes, and lepers, loving the unlovely and others commonly outcast by society as a model for a spiritual response to the struggles of persons with AIDS.

Body, mind, and spirit go together. Healing cannot occur, physical or spiritual, if anyone is left unattended. As occupational therapists, or as health care workers, clergy, caregivers, family members, or friends, we have a responsibility to respond to those hurt by AIDS. AIDS may not have a cure today, but despair has a cure. AIDS may lead to the discovery of the meaning and purpose in life so that a person's remaining days may be filled with promise and quality.

In the mean time,

> We must love each other through this—bearing one another's pain and affirming for each other the promise that neither death nor life; nor angels, nor principalities; neither things present, nor things to come; neither Kaposi's nor pneumocystis, nor any syndrome nor anguish nor pain, nor the hatred of those who fear us; nor anything else in all creation can separate us from the love of God or keep us from the kingdom prepared for us from the beginning of the world. (Fortunato, 1987. p. 89)

STUDY QUESTIONS

1. *In what sense is the person with HIV or AIDS on a spiritual journey?*
2. *As a caregiver, friend, or family member of a person with HIV or AIDS, what issues may your loved one deal with that may be spiritual in nature? How might you channel these toward healing?*
3. *What role does hope play in enhancing immune competency? Why is this important for the person with HIV or AIDS?*
4. *What does the term "spiritual" mean for you? Recall an experience in your life that was spiritually meaningful for you. What affect has it had on your life? What affect has it had on your thoughts about death?*
5. *What, personally, gives you hope? Why?*

REFERENCES

Amos, W. E., Jr. (1988). *When AIDS comes to church*. Philadelphia: Westminster Press.

Ayres, A. J. (1972). *Sensory integration and learning disorders*. Los Angeles: Western Psychological Services.

Bing, R. K. (1981). Occupational therapy revisited: A paraphrastic journey. *American Journal of Occupational Therapy, 35*, 499-518.

Bowers, C. C. (1987). Spiritual dimensions of the rehabilitation journey. *Rehabilitation Nursing, 12*, 90-1.

Cousins, N. (1979). *Anatomy of an illness*. New York: Bantam Books.

Cousins, N. (1983). *Human options*. New York: Berkley Books.

Cousins, N. (1989). *Head first: The biology of hope*. New York: E.P. Dutton.

D'Aloisio. S. (1989, February 23). For therapist treating AIDS patients, the best approach is to take each day as it comes. *OT Week*, p. 16-17.

Engelhardt, H. T., Jr. (1983). Occupational therapists as technologists and custodians of meaning. In G. Kielhofner (Ed.), *Health through occupation: Theory and practice in occupational therapy*. (pp.139-145). Philadelphia: F. A. Davis.

Farber, S. D. (1989). Neuroscience and occupational therapy: Vital connections. *American Journal of Occupational Therapy, 43*, 637-646.

Ferszt, G. G. & Taylor, P. B. (1988). When your patient needs spiritual comfort. *Nursing, 4*, 48-9.

Fortunato, J. E. (1987). *AIDS, the spiritual dilemma*. San Francisco: Harper and Row.

Garrett, J. E. (1988). The AIDS patient: Helping him and his parents cope. *Nursing, 18*, (9), 50-2.

Gaze, H. (1987). Keep morals out. *Nursing Times, 83*, (50), 31.

Haburchak, D., Harrison, S., Miles. F. W., & Hannon, R. N. (1989). Resolving patient feelings of guilt: A need for physician-chaplain liaison. *AIDS Patient Care, 3*, (5), 42-3.

Hamilton, D. (1988). For AIDS patients, the little things can mean a lot. *Nursing, 18*, (5), 61-2.

Hopkins, H. (1978). An historical perspective on occupational therapy. In H. Hopkins & H. Smith, (Eds.), *Willard and Spackman's occupational therapy* (fifth edition). (pp. 3-23). Philadelphia: J. B. Lippincott.

Johnson, D. W. (1981). *Reaching out: Interpersonal effectiveness and self actualization*. Englewood Cliffs, New Jersey: Prentice-Hall.

Jourard, S. M. (1964). *The transparent self*. New York: D. Van Nostrand.

Kubler-Ross, E. (1987). *AIDS: The ultimate challenge*. New York: Macmillan.

Marshall, T. A. (1987). Pastoral counseling: Care involves family and medical staff. *AIDS Patient Care, 1*, (2), 18-21.

Marshall, T. A. & Nieckarf, J. P. (1988). Bereavement counseling: Unique factors call for unique approaches. *AIDS-Patient Care, 2*, (2), 21-5.

McCaffrey, E. A. (1987). Counseling AIDS patients: Unique approach by Shanti therapists. *AIDS Patient Care, 1*, (2), 26-7.

Meyer, A. (1922). The philosophy of occupational therapy. *Archives of Occupational Therapy, 1*, 1-10.

Nelson, David L. (1988). Occupation: Form and performance. *American Journal of Occupational Therapy, 42*, 633-641.

Pizzi, M. (1988, August 18). Challenge of treating AIDS patients includes helping them lead functional lives. *OT Week*, pp. 6-7,31.

Pizzi, M. (1989). Occupational therapy: Creating possibilities for adults with HIV infection, ARC, and AIDS. *AIDS Patient Care, 3*, (1), 18-23.

Powell, J. (1978). *Unconditional love*. Allen, Texas: Argus Communications.

Scott, F. (1988, October 17). AIDS patients get helping hand in NY. OT Advance, pp. 12-13.

Shelp, E. E., Sunderland, R. H. & Mansell, P. W. (1986). *AIDS, personal stories in pastoral perspective*. New York: Pilgrim.

Simsen, B. (1988). Nursing the spirit. *Nursing Times, 84*, (37), 31-3.

Snow, J. (1987). *Mortal fear*. Cambridge, Massachusetts: Cowley.

Sharrot, G. W. (1983). Occupational therapy's role in the client's creation and affirmation of meaning. In G. Kielhofner (Ed.), *Health through occupation: Theory and practice in occupational therapy*. (pp. 213-235). Philadelphia: F. A. Davis.

Sodestrom, K. E. & Martinson, I. M. (1987). Patient's spiritual coping strategies: A study of nurse and patient perspectives. *Oncology Nursing Forum, 14*, (2), 41-6.

Tapia, A. (1988). *The AIDS crisis*. Downers Grove, IL: InterVarsity.

Vaillot, M. (1970). The spiritual factors in nursing. *Journal of Practical Nursing, 20*, (9), 30-1.

Weinstein, B. (1989, April). A holistic approach to AIDS. (Workshop presented at the American Occupational Therapy Association Annual Convention. Baltimore, MD.)

Yerxa, E. (1985). Authentic occupational therapy. In *A Professional legacy: The Eleanor Clarke Slagle lectures in occupational therapy, 1955-1984*. (pp. 155-173). Rockville, MD: American Occupational Therapy Association.

Infants and Children with HIV Infection: Perspectives in Occupational and Physical Therapy

Michael Pizzi, MS, OTR/L
Meredith Hinds-Harris, EdD, PT

SUMMARY. Infants and children with human immunodeficiency virus (HIV) infection are a rapidly growing population that can be viewed in the category of 'at risk.' These children and their families require rehabilitation services to facilitate adaptive responses to HIV infection. This article addresses the clinical manifestations of HIV infection and normal growth and development. The impact of HIV on growth and development is presented through a description of clinical interventions that highlight basic clinical need areas of children with HIV and their families. A rehabilitation classification system is introduced as a means to identify rehabilitation needs of children with HIV.

INTRODUCTION

HIV infection in children is not manifested in any one clinical picture in infants and children. Detection of the infection in infants usually occurs as a result of opportunistic infections which indicate immune system com-

---

Michael Pizzi is in private practice and is Health Care Consultant in chronic illness, hospice and AIDS. Address correspondence to the author at 8201 16th Street #1123, Silver Spring, MD 20910.

Meredith Hinds-Harris is in private practice and is Health Care Consultant in Metropolitan New York and Associate Professor, Department of Physical Therapy, Northeastern University, Boston, MA. The author may be contacted at 531 Main St., Rte. 130, Mashpee, MA 02649.

The first author gratefully acknowledges the contribution of Janice P. Burke, MA, OTR/L, for her assistance in the organization of this manuscript.

Both authors gratefully acknowledge the children and families with HIV infection they have been privileged to serve.

103

promise. Infants with HIV infection are then referred to therapists by a pediatrician or pediatric neurologist because of neurological and developmental deficits. Oftentimes, an undiagnosed infant is referred because of neurological and developmental abnormalities secondary to HIV rather than directly because of HIV infection.

HIV infection was considered to be rapidly fatal. Early research indicated a survival rate of six to twelve months post diagnosis. Now, with vigorous medical intervention for syndrome related fatal factors such as pneumocystis carinii pneumonia (PCP), other respiratory disorders, nutrition related disorders which may play a part in wasting syndromes, and the advent of promising drugs such as azidothymidine (AZT) and dideoxyinidine (DDI), prognosis has improved for some children. We now are beginning to see the effects of interventions which unmask chronic neurologic and developmental deficits and for which therapy interventions can be effective in improving the quality of life for children with HIV and their families.

BACKGROUND

Children acquire HIV through several routes of transmission. Falloon, Eddy, Roper and Pizzo (1988) describe blood product transfusion related infection during treatment for hemophilia or other coagulation disorders and sexual abuse as some routes of transmission. The primary mode of transmission is transplacentally or perinatally. This latter group comprises over 80% of the total number of infected infants and children (Institute of Medicine, 1988).

In the United States, mothers of these infected children acquire HIV through sexual intercourse with an infected person, through blood transfusion or through intravenous (IV) drug use. "Because such women are disproportionately Black or Hispanic, poor and urban, most infected children belong to such groups. In addition, most infected children (and infected women) are from New York, California, New Jersey or Florida, but the proportion of children from these areas is decreasing" (Falloon et al., 1988, p. 339). Post partum transmission via infected breast milk may also be possible, as suggested by the case of a breast fed infected child who had been born to a woman infected by post partum transfusion (Ziegler et al., 1985).

Current predictions estimate 10,000-20,000 HIV infected children by 1991, with the majority of those from Black and Hispanic cultures (Institute of Medicine, 1988). Currently, our health care system must prepare for the growth of this population and begin to identify necessary support services, such as occupational therapy (OT) and physical therapy (PT), that facilitate adaptive functioning for children with HIV and their caregivers.

CLINICAL MANIFESTATIONS

Children with HIV present a spectrum of clinical manifestations. These children may range from being asymptomatic to critically/terminally ill. Scott (1987) and Oleske (1987) describe a range of clinical manifestations (Table 1).

The time from infection to overt acquired immunodeficiency syndrome (AIDS) in children is shorter (1) in children than adults and (2) shorter in children infected perinatally than in those infected through transfusion (Rogers et al., 1987). Perinatally infected children have a median age at diagnosis of nine months, whereas children with transfusion acquired HIV have a median age at diagnosis of seventeen months (Rogers et al., 1987).

Falloon et al., (1988) describe several nonspecific manifestations (e.g., weight loss, low birth weight or failure to thrive, diarrhea, hepatosplenomegaly, dermatitis, fevers), bacterial infections (e.g., sepsis, pneumonia,

TABLE 1. Syndromes and Neurologic Findings in Children with HIV

Wasting Syndrome

Lymphoid Interstitial Pneumonitis

Recurrent Bacterial Infection

Lymphadenopathy Syndrome

Cardiomyopathy

Hepatitis

Renal Disease

Developmental Delay/Loss of Developmental Milestones

Chronic Encephalopathy

Seizure Disorders

Motor Dysfunction

Microcephaly

Abnormal CT Scan Findings - Cortical Atrophy, Calcifications meningitis), and opportunistic infections (e.g., PCP, disseminated cytomegalovirus, candida, disseminated mycobacterium avium intracellulare [MAI]). There is a four percent incidence of Kaposi's sarcoma (KS) noted in children with HIV; however KS is more common in adults, as are HIV-related lymphomas (Rogers et al., 1987).

The most common neurologic manifestation in children with HIV is encephalopathy. Encephalopathy can be the primary manifestation of HIV in children, resulting in developmental delay or in a deterioration of motor skills and cognitive functioning (Belman, 1985; Rubinstein, 1986; Epstein et al., 1986; Diamond, 1989). Neurologic abnormalities such as paresis, pyramidal tract signs, ataxia, abnormal tone or pseudobulbar palsy have been noted (Rubinstein, 1986). Microcephaly has been described in younger children (Epstein et al., 1986). Computerized tomographic (CAT) scans have shown cerebral atrophy and ventricular enlargement, calcification in the basal ganglia and frontal white matter (Belman et al., 1985; Epstein et al., 1986).

The clinical manifestations of HIV in infants and children, particularly encephalopathy, have a profound impact on normal growth and development. The arenas of reflex, motor, cognitive, social-emotional and play development are areas where OT and PT can have a profound impact on facilitating adaptive responses.

NORMAL GROWTH AND DEVELOPMENT

A child's interactions with both the physical and social environments begin at birth and can be described as playful and exploratory (Reilly, 1974). The fundamental tool of children for occupational and physical skill development is play. Among the skills children develop through play are personal activities of daily living (PADL). Underlying sensory-motor and cognitive abilities facilitate development of play, PADL and occupational roles. It is important for therapists to have a basic knowledge in normal growth and development in order to identify abnormal growth and development in children with HIV infection.

Reflex and Motor Development

Several theorists and clinicians identify a normal sequence of motor and reflex development (Gesell, 1940; Fiorentino, 1963; Bayley, 1965; Brazelton, 1973; Coley, 1978). Developmental charts and chronological scales assist therapists in identifying skill levels of children and chronologic and developmental levels according to current functional levels (Tables 2 and 3).

Cognitive Development

Jean Piaget (1959) is most noted for his development of cognitive theory (Table 4). Piaget views human beings as alert, interactive with the environment and able to process and interpret information, rather than be passive recipients of information. He views people as adaptive in nature through processes of assimilation and accommodation, whereby new information is processed by the mind changing in order to accommodate new experiences. Growth occurs through assimilation and accommodation.

Social-Emotional Development

Erikson (1975) focuses on psychosocial development via eight emotional stages or issues (Table 5). Each stage/issue in his theory must be resolved before proceeding adaptively to the next stage/issue. Erikson's developmental theory views human beings as interpersonal in nature, relating to the social and cultural environment through successful progression of his eight stages. How one achieves resolution of a particular issue hierarchically affects how one will deal with subsequent issues.

Play Development

Play is the most important activity in childhood. Play skill development and performance varies between children and age groups. Motor and psychosocial/emotional development and competence and mastery in the environment are developed through play (Florey, 1971; Michelman, 1971; Reilly, 1974; Robinson, 1977). Play function and dysfunction are examined through the domains of materials, action, people and settings (Takata, 1974; Behnke, 1982; Menarchek, 1982) (Table 6). Treatment goals and treatment are then designed around the need areas in each domain.

REHABILITATION EVALUATION
OF THE INFANT/CHILD WITH HIV

In order to appropriately develop OT/PT intervention, a holistic assessment of the child's functioning must be undertaken. Typical assessment strategies can include chart review, clinical observations, history taking,

TABLE 2. Reflex Development

Reflex	Approximate Age in months (normal response)
Primary Reflexes	
Rooting	0-3
Sucking	0-3
Moro	0-5
Galant	0-3
Palmar Grasp	0-3
Plantar Grasp	0-10
Crossed Extension	0-1
Primary Standing/Walking	0-2
Placing Reaction	0-6
Tonal Reflexes	
Asymmetrical tonic neck	0-6
Symmetrical tonic neck	0-12

Reflex	Approximate Age in Months (normal response)
Righting Reactions	
Labrynthine righting on head (prone)	0-life
Labrynthine righting on head (supine)	4-life
Landau	3-24
Body righting	4-life
Protective balance reactions	
Protective extension	6-life
Equilibrium reactions	
prone/supine	5-life
sitting	7-life

TABLE 3. Normal Growth and Development (motor)

Task	Developmental age
body lying prone	birth
body lying supine	birth
rolling side to side	1-4 weeks
rolling prone to supine	6 months
rolling supine to prone	7 months
propped sitting	6 months
sitting with hands propped	7 months
crawling all fours	7-8 months
standing	7-8 months
sitting unsupported	10-12 months
walking holding onto furniture	10 months
walking without support	10-12 months

developmental, play and ADL assessments, interviews of caregivers and standardized testing (Pizzi, 1989; Harris and Schlussel, 1989, June).

Neurodevelopmental assessment is a major part of the overall assessment of children with HIV. It is most important in children 0-5 years of age. A holistic assessment for therapists to explore includes the psychosocial and environmental (physical and social) domains of functioning. These domains, in concert with the domain of physical functioning, include the skills of play and selfcare.

CLINICAL INTERVENTIONS

In the population of children with HIV infection, important and different issues arise regarding intervention. Noteworthy are the issues of regression in skill performance, cultural considerations, caregivers who may also be coping with their own HIV disease, stigma, and environmental issues (most patients are poor urban dwellers with few economic or community resources) (Pizzi, 1989, April). Therefore, traditional treatment must be examined with regards to these population specific considerations.

TABLE 4. Piaget's Cognitive Development

Phase	Stage	Approximate Chronological Age
Sensorimotor	Reflexes, habits, circular reactions (primary, secondary, tertiary), deduction	0-2 years
Preoperational	Symbolism and imagery "magical thinking"	2-6 years
Concrete operational	Basic logic; inductive reasoning	6-12 years
Formal operational	Abstract thinking; deductive reasoning	12 years

Children with HIV may never achieve normal developmental milestones, or may develop slowly and/or experience loss of function. Therapists promote development of these milestones through neurodevelopmental treatment, positioning, adaptive equipment and play. Intervention with children with HIV must always include the family system and caregiver education (Pizzi, 1989).

Selfcare

Selfcare includes the areas of eating, bathing, grooming, hygiene, dressing, functional communication and mobility. Skills and established routines of daily living necessitate constant reassessment and adaptations due to the many complications and manifestations of HIV disease, such as motor and neurologic complications, frequent hospitalizations, psychoso-

TABLE 5. Social-Emotional Development – Erikson's Eight Stages

STAGE	AGES
Trust versus Mistrust	0-1
Autonomy versus Shame	1-3
Initiative versus Guilt	4-5
Industry versus Inferiority	6-11
Identity versus Role Diffusion	12-18
Intimacy versus Isolation	Young Adult
Generativity versus Stagnation	Middle Adult
Ego Integrity versus Despair	Later Adult

cial problems (e.g., poor self concept, self esteem or body image) and influence of caregivers on skill development. Treatment of selfcare must also include treatment and recognition of underlying clinical problems. Environmental and cultural influences on development of selfcare skills and routines must also be considered. For example, does the family's socioeconomic status interfere with function? Are there cultural considerations regarding use of utensils during mealtimes? Is the physical environment/physical space able to support selfcare, motor development and age appropriate play? Does the family system value selfcare independence for the child with HIV, or is it more important to develop other functional skills?

Adaptive Equipment and Strategies

Adaptive equipment and strategies to develop age appropriate selfcare and motor skills are often necessary. Children with HIV related neurologic manifestations require a structured environment and few distractions to accomplish tasks. For example, one command at a time (e.g., put legs into pants, pull up pants, zip up pants), using the same environment to perform daily living skills (e.g., child's room, bathroom) and having no one else around to distract the child with HIV related encephalopathy can help the child become more independent in dressing. Built up handles, plateguards, scoop dishes and velcro clothing are suggested for other selfcare needs. Adapted wheelchairs, seating and positioning can support caregivers in fostering independent selfcare function.

TABLE 6. Play Development

Sensorimotor (0-2 years)

Materials: Toys, objects for sensory experiences like rattles, balls, blocks, straddle toys, chimes, simple pictures, color cones, large blocks using sight, smell, hearing, touching and mouthing.

Action: Gross motor including stand/fall, walk, pull, sit on, climb, open/close. Fine motor including touch, mouthe, hold, throw/pick up, bang, shake, carry, motoric imitation of domestic actions.

People: Parents and immediate family.

Setting: Home - crib, playpen, floor, yard, immediate surroundings.

Emphasis is on independent play with exploration; habits expressed in trial and error.

Symbolic and Simple Constructive (2-4 years)

Materials: Toys, objects, raw materials (water, sand, paints, clay, crayon) for fine motor manipulation and simple combining and taking apart; wheeled vehicles and adventure toys to practice gross motor actions.

Action: Gross motor including climb, run, jump, balance, drag, dump, throw. Fine motor including empty/fill, scribble/draw, squeeze/pull, combine/take apart, arrange in spatial dimensions. Imagination with story telling; fantasy. Objects represent events and things.

People: Parents, peers and other adults.

Setting: Outdoors - playground or play equipment in immediate neighborhood. Indoors - home, nursery.

Emphasis is on parallel play and beginning to share. Symbolic play expressed in simple pretense and simple constructional use of materials.

Dramatic and Complex Constructive and Pre-Game (4-7 years)

Materials: Objects, toys, raw materials for fine motor actions and role-playing; large adventure toys for refining gross actions for speed and coordination; pets; nonselective collections.

Action: Gross motor including "daredevil" feats of hopping, skipping, turning somersaults, dance. Fine motor including combining materials and making products to do well, to use tools, to copy reality. Dramatic role-playing including imitating reality in part/whole costumes, story telling.

Dramatic and Complex Constructive and Pre-Game (CONT'D)

People: Peer group (2-5 members), imaginary friends, parents, immediate family, other adults.

Setting: School, neighborhood and extended surroundings (excursions), upper space and off the ground.

Emphasis is on cooperative play with purposeful use of materials for constructions; dramatization of reality and building habits of skill and tool use.

TABLE 6 (continued)

Games (7-12 years)

Materials: Games played with rules (dominoes, checkers,

table-card games, ping-pong); raw materials and

tools for making complex products (weaving,

woodwork, carving, needlework). Gross muscle sports

hopscotch, kite flying, skating, basketball.

Books--puzzles, "things to do', biography,

adventure, sports. Selective collection or hobby.

Pet.

Action: Gross motor including refining and combining skills

of jumping, hopping and running. Fine motor

including precision in using variety of tools, finer

object manipulation and construction. Making,

following and breaking rules; competition and

compromise with peers.

People: Peer group of same sex; organized group such as

scouts; parents; other adults

Setting: Neighborhood, playground, school, home.

Emphasis is on enhancement of constructional and sports skills

as expressed in rule-bound behavior, competition and

appreciation of process cooperative play.

Recreation (12-16 years)

Materials: Team games and sports and special interest groups

for music, dancing, singing, discussing.

Collections and hobbies; parties, books, table

games.

Action: Gross motor including team sports and individual

               precision sports (tennis and golf). Fine motor

               including applying and practicing fine manipulative

               skills to develop craftsmanship, special talents.

               Organized group work.

People: Peer group of same and opposite sex; parents and

               other adults.

Setting: School, neighborhood and extended community, home.

Emphasis is on team participation and independent action,

expressed in organized sports, interest groups and hobbies

during leisure time.

Play

Following the play taxonomy developed by Takata (1974), therapists make play recommendations to facilitate adaptive motor responses, including reflex and sensory integration, facilitate and inhibit tone, and facilitate exploratory behaviors and competence in the environment. Caregiver education on play and play development are crucial elements in treatment for children with HIV. Play recommendations, presented at the level of understanding of the caregiver, should be both written and oral to insure that caregivers understand the recommendations and their purpose (Pizzi, 1989).

Self Concept

Often, self-concept affects play and selfcare behaviors. Children with HIV, especially older children who have an understanding of the illness, can present clinically as withdrawn, anxious and noncommunicative. Children are also very perceptive and observe adult behaviors. From these behaviors they may sense they are 'different' or 'special.' Caregivers often state that there is a noted change in the child's play and that the child seems to 'mope around the house.' This psychosocial component can be addressed through interview with the caregiver and/or the child and through play observations. Intervention with a focus on activity produces successful outcomes and provides immediate positive feedback.

To help guide effective clinical interventions therapists also need information on the child's level of understanding of HIV and whether or not the child has been told the diagnosis and by whom. This information and knowledge of the child's behaviors prior to an HIV diagnosis can yield solid clinical data and support the patient-therapist relationship.

Psychosocial interventions include activities that are (1) short term, (2) of interest to the child, and (3) easily completed, and projects in which the child can be actively involved and feel good about that involvement and subsequent task achievement. An option is involvement in community projects, where the child makes a contribution to others and is acknowledged for the contribution (e.g., being a leader in developing a neighborhood carnival to raise money for charity or going to the store on a daily or weekly basis for an elder in the community) (Pizzi, 1989).

Physical Environment

Adaptations to the physical environment are also needed when children with HIV experience physical symptoms of HIV. The physical environment includes the home, school or playground. Children with HIV often have difficulties negotiating environments due to motor problems, diminished visual acuity and/or endurance problems. Adaptations to the physical environment can facilitate the child's active involvement in life activity and promote greater mobility. For example, a bedbound child can use a lap tray to hold books or write a paper or for leisure tasks while lying down.

An intercom or walkie-talkie can allow communication with others who may be in a different part of the house. Moving the child's bedroom to the most pleasant and active part of the house fosters ongoing communication and relationship within the family system. Ramps to accomodate wheelchairs can easily be built for the child at home and at school. Therapists can also be involved in adapting playgrounds in the child's community for the child with special needs.

Family System

The family system may be both parents, a single parent, a grandmother or even the pediatric unit of a hospital. It is often the family system that is responsible for on-going services, which requires their involvement in the rehabilitation process from the beginning of assessment through treatment. Families with HIV infected children often demonstrate and experience guilt, fear, anxiety, shame and grief.

Whether in denial or acceptance and understanding of HIV, the caregiver's reactions to HIV will affect the child and, hence, the child's functioning. Too, it has been noted clinically that the level of communication about the disease from caregiver to child affects function. For example, parents who were the only ones who knew the diagnosis of their child finally told their 10 year old son. Eventually, they told some community members and the church and were met, on the whole, with much support and outpouring of concern. The child began to experience a freedom from being 'special,' showed improvement psychosocially and played more interactively with friends (Pizzi, November 23, 1989).

The varying psychoemotional and physical functional levels of caregivers can impede or enhance the child's current and future functioning. This is especially true for caregivers who themselves are HIV positive or have AIDS. Caregivers who are symptomatic often must cope with musculoskeletal, neurologic and cardiopulmonary difficulties, as well as the physical and psychosocial needs of the HIV infected child and, if any, other siblings.

Therapists who provide therapy services to HIV infected infants, children and their families must be prepared to be flexible and adaptable in scheduling therapy sessions to meet the needs of the family as well as the child. Identification of an HIV infected child in a family is a window into a family system which is infected. Transmission from the mother to the infant prenatally or perinatally is the first indication that the mother is infected.

The sadness experienced in helping either natural or foster parents cope with the grief associated with having an HIV infected child is often ameliorated in occupational and physical therapy as hopefulness is engendered by the positive effects of touching, adaptation, holding and improving the child's quality of life. This may be noted through improving the quality of movement, feeding, breathing, playing and daily life skill management.

By teaching caregivers ways to hold, move, sit and play with their neurologically impaired children, a more positive bond is established. Parents sometimes feel these positive aspects are a welcome respite from coping with the bouts of illness and trips to emergency rooms that are an inherent part of the medical emergencies which frequently arise. Currently, a Family Assessment of Occupational Functioning (FAOF), developed by three occupational therapists, is in the initial stages of research to address occupational needs and behaviors of family systems (Pizzi, 1989, November).

A PEDIATRIC HIV CLASSIFICATION SYSTEM

Questions arise about when to intervene with OT/PT, how to best schedule the frequency and duration of therapy and how to educate natural and foster families, other care givers, teachers, social workers, and social service agencies about the need and efficacy of therapy intervention. There are various times in the course or progression of HIV associated disorders when intensive therapy is warranted. There are other times when periodic evaluation, monitoring and parent or school education and training is more appropriate. Sadly, there are also times when parents and therapist must decide that therapy is a low priority when keeping therapy appointments creates additional stress too great for the family or it exceeds the child's energy levels.

Longitudinal follow-up of large numbers of children has permitted categorization of several neurological courses in pediatric HIV infection (Belman, 1985) but the course of any one child is determined only with careful, consistent, standardized documentation and longitudinal follow-up. Information from diagnostic tests and clinical reports help identify the clinical course of the disease and understanding of the underlying pathology. Belman (1985) reported six categories of neurological progression based on a study of six children. These categories have been further expanded by Harris and Schlussel (1989, June), based on their clinical experiences. They are defined as follows:

1. rapidly progressive;
2. subacute relentlessly progressive;
3. subacute progressive with plateau;
4. static encephalopathy;
5. moderately impaired neurological course;
6. mild to moderate deficits;
7. mildly impaired neurological course; and
8. normal mental and motor neurological course.

Each category is described below.

Rapidly Progressive

The infant is identified with HIV infection within the first few months after birth, has frequent opportunistic infections and rapidly progressive neurological deterioration with a poor prognosis. Death usually occurs within six months to two years after initial diagnosis.

Subacute Relentlessly Progressive

The infant may be severely deficient with neurologic deterioration which begins insidiously and progresses at an individually determined rate for each child.

Subacute Progressive with Plateau

Progression of deterioration may be slow and marked by periodic plateaus.

Static Encephalopathy

The child is relatively stable medically, but has moderate to severe deficits in any of the following areas: gross and fine motor developmental milestone achievement; sensory, behavioral and functional skills; automatic reactions and speech. Evidence suggests that encephalopathy results from HIV infection in the central nervous system (CNS), probably in utero (Falloon et al., 1988).

The route and timing of HIV CNS invasion and the pathogenic mechanism are uncertain. The course may be marked by global developmental, motor and cognitive deficits which may be in evidence at birth or may not develop until later in the first year of life. This child has moderate to severe deficits in motor development, automatic reactions, developmental milestone achievement, language and cognition, feeding, tonal disorders, paresis and respiration. At the time of evaluation, these children may be in a plateau or may demonstrate static encephalopathy. Age may vary from 10 months to three years.

Categories 2, 3, and 4 are grouped together because it is difficult to determine whether changes seen in the child are a result of the progressive disease process or whether the factors identifying them permit misclassification. These children may alternate between categories. For example, when first seen for evaluation, a child may present with what appears to be static encephalopathy, deteriorates over the course of treatment, and then responds to treatment as deterioration slows. This course is marked by severe developmental, cognitive and neurological deficits with frequent increasingly severe acute illnesses.

Moderately Impaired Neurological Course

The child in this category is characterized by moderate deficits in motor, perceptual, sensory, cognitive and behavioral areas. Health is impaired by different and frequent mild infections, high fevers of undetermined origin, chronic repiratory disorders, and asymptomatic lymphadenopathy. These medical problems may require frequent trips to the emergency room or frequent absences from school but are not severe enough to warrant long term hospitalization nor do they leave the child with residual impairment or loss of achieved skills.

Mild to Moderate Deficits

This category includes children who have mild to moderate deficits in fine and gross motor, behavioral, sensory and/or social areas. Children in this category may not be in need of specific physical and occupational therapy but may benefit from small group multidisciplinary early intervention programs. Because of the potential for insidious deterioration, children who are identified with HIV and who have relatively mild symptoms should be evaluated periodically as ninety percent of these children develop neurological and/or cognitive deficits and loss of developmental milestones and functional skills over time. Some indications of neurological deterioration include an abrupt change in tone with an appearance or increase of spasticity, particularly in the lower extremities; an increase in abdominal or extensor tone; a decrease in postural tone in the trunk; loss of tone in the upper extremities, behavioral change (sometimes a generalized apathy); loss of functional skills or loss of automatic postural reactions. Other indications of deterioration include clumsiness and increasingly frequent falls, changes in eating or feeding patterns, alternating periods of constipation, and diarrhea.

The sometimes rapid onset of spasticity or rigidity which quickly progresses to contractures and subsequent loss of function as well as a loss of motor milestones is frustrating for the therapist, child and caregiver. The psychological impact on the child of skill loss can be devastating. Acute illness associated with deterioration precludes therapeutic intervention. There are times when parents should endeavor to keep therapy appointments for the child in order to prevent contractures and rapid loss of function. Therapy includes facilitation of movement, prevention of contractures, facilitation of automatic reactions and provision of adaptive equipment and positioning to continue function. The quality of life for the child and the family may be enhanced by intervention and by providing positive goals even in periods of deterioration.

Therapists treating an undiagnosed child should be alert to indications of deterioration, including abrupt changes in tone, appearance of primitive reflexes not previously in evidence, loss of developmental milestones, developmental plateaus, chronic respiratory or other infections from opportunistic pathogens, loss of feeding skills, and a progressive generalized apathy. These symptoms are by no means conclusive indications of HIV infection or AIDS but may alert the therapist to refer the child for medical workup to rule out progressive neurological diseases.

The importance of an accurate evaluation and clear documentation of therapy outcomes become critical in identifying changes that occur over time.

Mildly Impaired Neurological Course

Similar but milder deficits as in category 5.

Normal Mental and Neurological Course

Children with no mental or motor deficits are referred to OT and PT from physicians for baseline evaluation. They need no specific intervention at the time they are seen. They also may be seen for acute care of respiratory and ear infections or skin rashes; because they are relatively asymptomatic, they are not in need of physical or occupational therapy interventions.

Repeated periodic evaluations on specific measures help determine the areas in which change is occurring. These clinical signs may be the first indication of symptoms or may signal deterioration.

Categories five through eight are now becoming apparent as a result of longitudinal follow-up. Children representative of these groups may not have been identified until preschool age or later and may have previously been asymptomatic. They later develop neurological signs or opportunistic infections which may require reclassification as time elapses and neurological deficits occur with disease progression. Some children in these groups previously may have been identified as static encephalopathy. They also may have had acute illnesses and other signs of HIV infection, such as lymphadenopathy, and demonstrate slow subtle deterioration, if any, in motor or mental status.

Depending on when the child is referred or identified as needing therapy services, the exact neurological course is undetermined until HIV infection status is first identified. The child is then followed with careful documentation of neurological and developmental progress or regression.

CONCLUSION

This article has presented an overview of normal growth and development and the impact of HIV infection on infants, children and their families. Clinical interventions from the perspective of occupational and physical therapy have been described, noting that holistic assessment and treatment must include the family system as the unit of care. A pediatric

HIV classification system has been described to assist therapists in developing timely and appropriate clinical interventions.

REFERENCES

Belman, A., Ultmann, M.H. and Houroupian, D. (1985). Neurological complications in infants and children with acquired immunodeficiency syndrome. *Annals of Neurology, 18,* 560-566.

Bayley, N. (1965). Comparisons of mental and motor test scores for age 1-15 months by sex, birthorder, race, geographic location and education of parents. *Child Development, 36,* 379-411.

Brazelton, T.B. (1973). *Neonatal behavior assessment scale.* Philadelphia: J.B. Lippincott Co.

Coley, I.L. (1978). *Pediatric assessment of selfcare activities.* St. Louis: C.V. Mosby.

Diamond, G.W. (1989). Developmental problems in children with HIV infection. *Mental Retardation, 27*(4), 213-217.

Epstein, L.G., Sharer, L.R. and Oleske, J.M. (1986). Neurological manifestations of HIV infection in children. *Pediatrics, 78,* 678-687.

Erikson, E.H. (1975). *Eight ages of man: Life the continuous process.* New York: Alfred A. Knopf, Inc.

Falloon, J., Eddy, J., Roper, M. and Pizzo, P. (1988). AIDS in the pediatric population. In DeVita, V., Hellman, S. and Rosenberg, T. (Eds.), *AIDS: Etiology, diagnosis, treatment and prevention* (pp. 339-351). Philadelphia: J.B. Lippincott Co.

Fiorentino, M. (1963). *Reflex testing methods for evaluating CNS development (2nd edition; 2nd printing).* Springfield, Illinois: Charles C Thomas.

Florey, L. (1971). An approach to play and play development. *American Journal of Occupational Therapy, 25*(6), 275-280.

Gesell, A. (1940). *The first five years of life.* New York: Harper and Row.

Harris-Copp, M. (1988). The HIV infected child: A critical need for physical therapy. *Clinical Management in Physical Therapy,* 8(1).

Harris-Copp, M. and Schlussel, S. (1989, June). Paper presented for the conference "Children, AIDS and Developmental Disabilities: A Challenge for the 1990's." New York City.

Michelman, S. (1971). The importance of creative play. *American Journal of Occupational Therapy, 25*(6), 285-290.

Oleske, J.M. (1987). Natural history of HIV infection II. In *Report of the Surgeon General's Workshop on Children with HIV Infection and Their Families.* United States Department of Health and Human Services.

Piaget, J. (1954). *The construction of reality in the child.* New York: Basic Books, Inc.

Pizzi, M. (1989, April). Pediatric AIDS. Workshop presented at the Annual Conference of the American Occupational Therapy Association. Baltimore, Maryland.

Pizzi, M. (1989, November). AIDS and Rehabilitation: The Caregiver and Their Needs. Paper presented at the Annual Conference of the American Congress of Rehabilitation Medicine. San Antonio, Texas.

Pizzi, M. (1989, November 23). Pediatric AIDS: Occupational therapy assessment and treatment. *OT Week*, pp. 6-7, 10.

Pizzi, M. (1989). Occupational therapy: Creating possibilities for children with HIV infection, ARC, and AIDS. *AIDS Patient Care*, December, 31-36.

Robinson, A.L. (1977). Play: The arena for aquisition of rules for competent behavior. *American Journal of Occupational Therapy*, *31*(4), 248-253.

Rogers, M.F., Thomas, P.A., and Starcher, E.T. (1987). Acquired immunodeficiency syndrome in children: Report of the Centers for Disease Control national surveillance, 1982-1985. *Pediatrics*, *79*, p. 1008.

Rubinstein, A. (1986). Pediatric AIDS. *Current Problems in Pediatrics*, *16*, 361.

Scott, G. (1987). Natural history of HIV infection in children. In *Report of the Surgeon General's Workshop on Children with HIV Infection and Their Families*. United States Department of Health and Human Services.

Takata, N. (1974). Play as a prescription. In M. Reilly (Ed.), *Play as Exploratory Learning* (pp. 209-246). Beverly Hills, CA: Sage Publications.

Tower, G. (1983). Selected developmental reflexes and reactions: A literature search. In H.L. Hopkins and H.D. Smith (Eds.), *Willard and Spackman's Occupational Therapy* (6th Edition) (pp. 175-187). Philadelphia: J.B. Lippincott.

Ziegler, J.B., Cooper, D.A. and Johnson, R.O. (1985). Postnatal transmission of AIDS associated retrovirus from mother to infant. *Lancet*, 896.

Occupational Therapy: Creating Possibilities for Adults with Human Immunodeficiency Virus Infection, AIDS Related Complex, and Acquired Immunodeficiency Syndrome

Michael Pizzi, MS, OTR/L

SUMMARY. Occupational therapists prevent dysfunction and maintain and restore function for people with HIV/AIDS in the areas of work, selfcare and play/leisure. These occupational areas are assessed and treated from psychosocial, physical and environmental perspectives. This article examines occupational therapy assessment and treatment for people with HIV/AIDS with the primary focus on adaptive equipment, energy conservation, habits and time management, and work.

INTRODUCTION

Annie is 27 years old and married with four children. Before the birth of her fourth child, she became much more fatigued than she remembered when she had her other children. She often could not get out of bed until noon, and to cook, clean and care for her husband and children seemed nearly impossible. She also took in extra homemaking tasks and two other children to earn extra money. Her husband, a laborer, became forgetful at work, belligerent at others more often than usual, and would often miss

Michael Pizzi is in private practice and is Health Care Consultant in chronic illness, hospice and AIDS.

This article is adapted and reprinted from AIDS Patient Care, Vol. 3, No. 1, February, 1989, Mary Ann Liebert, Inc., Publishers, 1651 Third Ave., New York, New York, 10128. Used with permission.

work. Seven months after the fourth child was born, Annie still noticed great fatigue and some forgetfulness. She also noticed that her child could not hold his head up, had a fixed gaze and could not smile. After seeing a pediatrician, and having the baby tested for HIV, she was told the baby was seropositive. She also was found to be positive. Her husband refused testing but soon thereafter admitted to an intravenous (IV) drug habit. He died two months later.

John is a successful 38 year old businessman. He owns three beauty shops, a health club and two restaurants. He and his partner of twelve years, Bill, enjoy participating in sports and going to the health club to work out daily. Cooking and gardening are favorite pasttimes, but John has little time to give to them. John views himself as a "workaholic." He derives great satisfaction from his work and from being physically fit and looking good. At the health club one day, he noted a small purplish mark on his right calf and could not scrub it off in the shower. He denied its seriousness until he was later hospitalized with pneumocystis carinii pneumonia (PCP) as well as Kaposi's sarcoma. He lost interest in exercising and in his work. He would stay home and watch TV, an activity he despised but accepted as 'something to do.' His weight and appearance altered considerably. He began to make demands on his partner, and his partner finally left, unable to cope with role changes seen in John and his own seropositivity. Friends would visit less often due to John's anger and continuous frustration at not being able to do favored activities. John could not accept the support of others very easily, being a very independent person. He felt helpless, hopeless and, despite past successes, felt life had no meaning any longer. Although he now had time to cook and garden, he refused to do so, stating "What's the use?"

These case scenarios are very real and occur daily. They touch upon a very real aspect of human functioning—life activity and the meaning it has for individuals. People with human immunodeficiency virus (HIV) infection, AIDS Related Complex (ARC) and acquired immunodeficiency syndrome (AIDS) often experience, at some level, an alteration in life activity.

How can one be taught to cope with the many physical, psychosocial and environmental changes experienced during the course of an illness? How does one regain skills or improve human functioning despite illness? How can people with HIV and AIDS, their families and significant others be empowered to maintain function—performing life activities of choice, interest and those unique to one's value system—in the face of a chronic illness? Occupational therapy provides some answers.

OCCUPATIONAL THERAPY AND ITS MISSION

The roots of occupational therapy can be traced back to treatment approaches used in nineteenth century psychiatry. Treatment consisted of normal activities carried out in an environment supportive of daily living occupations to promote meaningful involvement in life and included the belief that patients needed kind and compassionate care (Bockoven, 1972; Pizzi, 1987b).

A sense of community was established by having people engage in daily living occupations together. Occupations included manual work, intellectual work, recreation and worship. Work, play and social activities, when carefully applied and structured to balance one's day and time, succeeded at producing a meaningful total life experience (Bockoven, 1972).

In the early 1920s, Adolph Meyer, a psychiatrist, created a paradigm of occupation, which later became the profession of occupational therapy. It was holistic in scope. Meyer, and later others in the profession, recognized that: (1) an individual's health is measured by involvement in life tasks in the social and physical environments; (2) focus must be on a person's lifestyle; (3) there must be a healthy balance between work, rest, sleep and play in order to fully function; (4) occupations (daily living activities) can restore and maintain function and prevent dysfunction; (5) occupations assist one in making better use of time and in reorganizing time (Kielhofner, 1986).

From the early twentieth century to the present time, occupational therapy has been a profession with a humanitarian approach, focusing on life activity and the 'doing' process of living. Now and into the next century, occupational therapy has an obligation to bring humanitarian and compassionate treatment to the lives of people with HIV and AIDS. Occupational therapy can provide people with HIV and AIDS the means by which independent productive living can be maintained, despite progressive chronic illness. When independent productive living is achieved, a sense of dignity and self-respect is maintained.

OCCUPATIONAL THERAPY EVALUATION FOR THE AIDS PATIENT

It is the author's contention that every person with HIV and AIDS should have an occupational therapy evaluation. Occupational therapists are found in most general hospitals and rehabilitation centers, and services are usually provided by local visiting nurse associations (VNA). A physician referral is needed for occupational therapy evaluation and treatment.

Anyone can request occupational therapy services, for oneself or for others, by calling the local VNA, home health agency or by making a request to the primary care physician. Payment for occupational therapy services varies between states.

Evaluation tools are designed as a battery of tests. This battery comprehensively determines the overall needs of people with HIV and AIDS. A detailed assessment battery can be found in Table 1. Evaluation encompasses the areas of functioning in the physical, psychosocial and environmental domains of life.

Human beings cannot be separated from their interaction with the environment, be it a social, physical (home, work, school) or cultural environment. Mind, body and spirit can also never be separated. Thus, it is essential that evaluation encompass all of these areas, using a mind, body, environment interactional framework.

As noted in Table 1, the evaluation tools are listed under several headings. These headings are areas of human functioning that act together to create what is called occupation, or occupational behaviors. Human functioning can be viewed from this Model of Human Occupation (Kielhofner and Burke, 1980) (see Table 2).

Volition enacts and guides choices of action. (I choose to play tennis because I feel competent at it, I am interested in playing twice a week and it is a meaningful activity to me.) Habituation maintains action through habits, which are behaviors or actions that are routine, something done regularly or unconsciously. (I wake at 6:30 to the alarm every morning, I dress, shave, eat, and go to work). Roles are how one defines oneself and provide a sense of identity (e.g., hobbyist, worker, student, home maintainer, friend, family member). The performance subsystem consists of skills that produce action (e.g., a combination of muscles, nerves, thought processes and communication skills that allow one to pick up a tennis racket, cook a meal, or rise to get to work on time). As the reader can see, human functioning and life activity (occupation) are more than just action.

OCCUPATIONAL THERAPY TREATMENT OF PEOPLE WITH AIDS

People with HIV and AIDS experience multiple occupational changes of habits, roles, and skills throughout the course of illness, mostly as a direct result of progressive signs and symptoms. These signs and symptoms can include fatigue, severe weight loss, neuropathy, encephalopathy (dementia), and Kaposi's sarcoma (Institute of Medicine, 1986). Occupational therapists evaluate and treat all areas of human functioning through-

TABLE 1. Assessment Battery for Adults with HIV

Component	Assessment
	VOLITION
Personal Causation	Occupational History (Moorehead, 1969)
	Occupational Questions (Pizzi, in
	Munknd, in press)
	Psychological Adjustment to Illness
	Scale (Morrow, Ciarello, and
	Derogatis, 1978)
	Locus of Control (Rotter, 1966)
Values	Occupational History
	Occupational Questions
	Role Checklist (Oakley, Kielhofner,
	Barris and Reichler, 1986)
	Time Reference Inventory (Roos and
	Albers, 1965)
	Psychological Adjustment to Illness
	Scale
Interests	Occupational History
	Occupational Questions
	Psychological Adjustment to Illness
	Scale

TABLE 1 (continued)

HABITUATION

Roles	Occupational History
	Occupational Questions
	Role Checklist
	Psychological Adjustment to Illness Scale
Habits	Occupational History
	Occupational Questions
	Psychological Adjustment to Illness Scale
	Activity Record*
	Interview

PERFORMANCE

Skills	Occupational History
	Occupational Questions
	Activities of Daily Living
	Activity Record
	Clinical Observations/Biomedical Assessment
Environment	Occupational History
	Occupational Questions
	Home Assessments
	Pizzi Social Environment Interview (Pizzi, in press)

TABLE 1 (continued)

* Available from Gloria Furst, MPH, OTR/L, National Institutes

of Health, Occupational Therapy Service, 6th Floor, Clinical

Center, 9000 Rockville Pike, Bethesda, MD 20892

** Available from the Occupational Therapy Service, National

Institutes of Health, 9000 Rockville Pike, 6th Floor, Clinical

Center, Bethesda, MD 20892

out the course of illness. Treatments are tailored to the individual, given that each person's life activity and life experience is unique. Treatments are primarily in the form of adaptation and recommendations for occupation.

TREATMENT SPECIFICS

Adaptive Equipment/Strategies

Often, individuals with AIDS will experience great fatigue, sensory changes in the hands and feet (neuropathy), dementia, and even damage to the spinal cord, resulting in physical impairment. Occupational therapists are skilled in evaluating needs for adaptive equipment and strategies to maintain and improve function. One who experiences fatigue during activity may use a tub seat, guard rails for safety, and adaptive strategies like sitting versus standing during selfcare activities (e.g., bathing and dressing). People with neuropathy may require built-up handles on utensils, adaptive cups, velcro and special adaptive equipment to button, zip, hold and carry objects. Also, equipment is available to improve writing, turn pages on a book, cook, clean, and other daily activities that are specific to the individual who may have problems using one's hands or standing for long periods of time.

People with dementia usually require adaptive strategies that include developing a structured way to remember items or routine tasks. Writing things or having visual or auditory reminders in the home or workplace assists in recall. In later stages of dementia, keeping familiar environments (e.g., home, one's room) clutter free, but with the same furniture arrangements, can reduce frustration for the person with dementia and provide a safe and negotiable area.

TABLE 2. The Model of Human Occupation*

ENVIRONMENT

VOLITION

  Personal Causation

    Belief in skill

    Belief in efficacy of skill

    Expectancy of success/failure

    Internal/external control

  Values

    Temporal orientation

    Meaningfulness of activity

    Occupational goals

    Personal standards

  Interests

    Discrimination

    Pattern

    Potency

HABITUATION

  Roles

    Perceived incumbency

    Internalized expectations

    Balance

  Habits

    Degree of organization

    Social appropriateness

    Flexibility/rigidity

```
PERFORMANCE

  Skills

    Interpersonal/communication

    Process

    Perceptual motor skill constituents

      Symbolic

      Neurological

      Musculoskeletal
```

* (Kielhofner and Burke, 1980)

Energy Conservation

Many people with HIV and AIDS experience fatigue, may develop cardiac complications, neuropathies and have muscle wasting, thus diminishing physical capacity to carry out daily living tasks. Conserving energy so that one can engage in performing life tasks that one enjoys (e.g., social activities, shopping, gardening) and not wasting energy in tasks that are routine (e.g., showering, dressing) can be very important. Some specific energy conservation suggestions include sitting rather than standing to dress, bathe or carry out other activities like cooking, cleaning or lecturing; preparing all equipment one needs before performing a task (e.g., setting out all utensils needed for a meal and then sitting to prepare the meal); having equipment used on a routine basis more readily accessible in cabinets and closets (e.g., in lower cabinets, on shelves).

Habits/Time Management

From the time we get up until the time we go to sleep, we engage in a specific routine of doing things and managing our time. People with HIV and AIDS, due to the variability of the illness with daily changing of activity patterns, usually require intervention for reestablishing productive habits and routines of daily living and developing activity/time management skills to cope with their changing medical condition. The balance of work, rest, sleep and play often is disrupted when one can no longer work or engage in meaningful activity. Restructuring habits and normalizing routines, commensurate with a person's interests, choices, values, roles and needs, is essential (Pizzi, 1987a).

Some specific questions an occupational therapist may ask are: (a) What times of day are best for you? When do you feel most/least productive? What activities create more/less fatigue and frustration?; (b) Have you given up a certain favored activity and changed the way you perform other activities? Why? Do you want to change this?; (c) Does it take longer or shorter periods of time to do certain activities (e.g., two hours to bathe and dress versus twenty minutes)?; (d) Do you still work? If not, how do you stay productive during the day? How do you fill your time? Would you change it if you could?; (e) Does pain, fatigue, sadness or depression prevent you from carrying out your daily routine?

Habit retraining examines more than time use. This is a critical area of care and intervention that occupational therapists use to prevent physical and psychosocial breakdown and to help people adapt to changes in their activity and daily routine.

Work

Ninety-eight percent of reported cases of HIV infection, ARC and AIDS are people in the worker years, ages 20 to 60 (Pizzi, 1988, August). This statistic is expected to remain constant for many years. A majority of people who experience AIDS related symptoms and/or who have full blown AIDS have difficulty at work due to inability to continue to produce and/or discrimination and subsequent job loss. When people no longer work, there are major implications. People often lose necessary health benefits and the financial picture becomes bleak. Most importantly, and a fact that many employers, individuals and even society can easily overlook, is that people often lose a sense of security, pride and self-esteem as they are no longer involved in an aspect of work that is vital to human functioning—being productive. Given that people work for a number of reasons, it is vital that the occupational therapist evaluate those reasons and plan treatment according to an individual's choices, interests and values.

Adapted work strategies can be implemented after the occupational therapist and person with HIV (and sometimes the significant other) create goals together around the work issue. Some specific suggestions include the following.

1. Looking at and writing down the reasons one works. What is the first thing on the list? How does it feel to have or not have that now? Have the person do a self-analysis of the list and ask "Is this really true for me and can I still have this by doing something other than the work I do or did?" Has the list changed since one was diagnosed and over the course of time?

2. If being productive is valuable, how can one plan to manage time in productive ways to replace work.

3. Has the person communicated to his/her employer the desire to work part-time, change job function or consult in order to maintain a work role and be productive? Have the person look at the possibilities if full time work is no longer feasible.

4. Is the person a 'workaholic?' Is work still that valuable? What makes it so valuable that one feels the need to work so many hours? Is the person avoiding or denying something by working so much?

5. Are there recreational or other work pursuits the person has wanted to try and did not or could not? Does the person have the time and interest to do those now? Have the person make a list, select some and incorporate them into a new daily routine (Pizzi, 1988).

Some people with HIV and AIDS have never worked and may never work. However, other roles may be developed that can be productive and not necessarily work related. An example is to develop time in one's schedule to volunteer at a hospital or community organization. The person with HIV and AIDS can make a contribution to other human beings, which is a very valuable and productive role in our society.

Other Treatments

Occupational therapists utilize a variety of strategies to prevent dysfunction and improve/maintain function in work, selfcare and play/leisure. Some other general treatment strategies can include biofeedback and relaxation training, occupations to improve physical functioning, occupations to improve self esteem and self concept, strategies to help individuals and loved ones cope with occupational role transitions, and strategies to help individuals and loved ones deal and cope with grief, loss and death and dying.

CONCLUSION

People with HIV and AIDS, and all human beings, require kind and compassionate care and consideration of their individuality and uniqueness. Occupational therapy is grounded in these beliefs. Through occupation one's strengths and possibilities for life and living can be realized. Despite chronic illness one can still be a productive human being. Occupational therapy can help people with HIV and AIDS maintain productivity throughout the lifespan, can transform impossibilities to possibilities, and can change disability to ability.

REFERENCES

Bockoven, J.S., (1972). *Moral treatment in community mental health*. New York: Springer Publishing Co.

Institute of Medicine, (1986). *Confronting AIDS: Directions for public health, health care and research*. Washington, DC: National Academy Press.

Kielhofner, G., (1985). *A Model of Human Occupation: Theory and application*. Baltimore: Williams and Wilkins.

Kielhofner, G. and Burke, J.P., (1980). A Model of Human Occupation, part 1: Conceptual framework and content. *American Journal of Occupational Therapy*, 34, 572-581.

Moorehead, L., (1969). The occupational history. *American Journal of Occupational Therapy*, 23, 329-334.

Morrow, G., Ciarello, R. and Derogatis, L., (1978). A new scale for assessing patients psychosocial adjustment to medical illness. *Psychological Medicine*, 8, 605-610.

Oakley, F., Kielhofner, G., Barris, R., and Reichler, R., (1986). The Role Checklist: Development and empirical assessment of reliability. *Occupational Therapy Journal of Research*, 6, 157-170.

Pizzi, M., (1987a). *Terminal care: A holistic and humanitarian approach*. Unpublished master's project, Towson State University, Towson, MD.

Pizzi, M., (1987b). *Challenges and opportunities for caregivers of people with AIDS*. Paper presented at the National Institutes of Health, Bethesda, MD.

Pizzi, M., (1988). *AIDS and occupational therapy*. Paper presented for the New York University AIDS Project, New York, New York.

Pizzi, M., (1988, August 18). Challenge of treating AIDS patients includes helping them lead functional lives. *OT Week*, pp. 6-7, 31.

Pizzi, M., (in press). Occupational therapy: Creating possibilities for children with HIV infection, ARC and AIDS. *AIDS Patient Care*.

Pizzi, M., (in press). HIV infection and occupational therapy. In John Munknd, (Ed.), AIDS and rehabilitation. New York: McGraw-Hill.

Roos, P. and Albers, R., (1965). Performance of alcoholics and normals on a measure of temporal orientation. *Journal of Clinical Psychology*, 21, 34-36.

Rotter, J., (1966). Generalized expectancies for internal versus external control of reinforcement. *Psychological Monograph*, 80, 1-28.

Scaffa, M., (1981) *Temporal adaptation and alcoholism*. Unpublished master's thesis. Virginia Commonwealth University, Richmond, Virginia.

APPENDIX A. Resources for Adaptive Equipment

Comfortably Yours

61 West Hunter Avenue

Maywood, NJ 07607

Enrichments for Better Living

Enrichments, Inc.

145 Tower Drive

P.O. Box 579

Hinsdale, Illinois 60521

Ableware: Independent Living from Maddak, Inc.

Pequannock, NJ 07440-1993

201-694-0500

Sears, Roebuck and Co.

Healthcare Merchandise Catalog

3333 W. Athington Street

Chicago, Illinois 60607

(or call local Sears store)

American Occupational Therapy Association

1383 Piccard Dr. P.O. Box 1725

Rockville, MD 29850-4375

301-948-9626

Psychosocial Issues
of Children and Families
with HIV/AIDS

Marcy Kaplan, MSW, LCSW

SUMMARY. The complex psychosocial issues for families who have a child diagnosed with HIV infection present a series of unique challenges for all health care providers. All members of the interdisciplinary team must be knowledgeable about these factors in providing all aspects of care to the child within the context of the family unit. Fear and secrecy are at the core of all persons living with HIV and AIDS, and health care providers must respond with compassion, empathy and sensitivity. The issues that will be discussed address the multiple factors that most frequently impact on a family's ability to function following their child's diagnosis of HIV infection or clinical AIDS and through the bereavement process. Concerns related to school attendance and the use of community services will be highlighted.

INTRODUCTION

Nationwide, 1,947 children under the age of thirteen have been diagnosed with Acquired Immunodeficiency Syndrome (AIDS) (Centers for Disease Control, November, 1989). This number does not reflect the number of children with Human Immunodeficiency Virus (HIV) who do not meet the Center for Disease Control (CDC) guidelines for an AIDS diagnosis. Authorities suggest that the actual number of children infected with HIV is approximately three times the number of CDC reported cases

Marcy Kaplan is Project Manager of the Los Angeles Pediatric AIDS Network. Ms. Kaplan was directly involved in the psychosocial care of children with HIV and their families from 1985-88 as the Clinical Social Worker and Program Coordinator of the Pediatric AIDS Program at Childrens Hospital, Los Angeles and predict that by the year 1991 there will be over 3000 children with AIDS in the United States (Koop, 1987).

Clearly, in lieu of the rapidly growing number of children who will be receiving treatment for HIV related problems, health care providers will need to be well versed in the many psychosocial issues that will have an impact on families. The following discussion will present an overview of the social characteristics of families with HIV, implications for health care providers, the psychosocial features encountered, strategies for intervention, and concerns pertaining directly to the child who is HIV infected.

Since the first case of reported childhood HIV infection in 1982, social workers as well as other health care providers have continually been challenged by the features that set HIV and AIDS apart from other chronic illnesses and public health problems. Although our ultimate goal is to view HIV as other chronic, long-term diseases are viewed, this is clearly not the case at the present time.

Due to the stigma attached to all individuals diagnosed with HIV-related diseases, and because of the atrocities that have been experienced following the disclosure that one has HIV, most individuals do not share this information with anyone. Consequently, they live in a world of secrecy and fear. Living in fear of social abandonment, families who have a child diagnosed with HIV infection continually grapple with decisions. While wanting desperately to give their families some semblance of normalcy, they must also act in the best interests of a child diagnosed with HIV infection. These goals are frequently incompatible and create additional stress on the family unit. Additionally, many of these issues affect health care providers who constantly deal with ethical and legal dilemmas and work closely with the child and family who must cope with HIV or AIDS.

THE HEALTH CARE TEAM

Although health care professionals generally have defined roles within the context of the interdisciplinary team structure, it is important that each has a comprehensive understanding of all aspects of HIV infection. Unlike health care teams working closely with children with chronic illnesses, such as cancer or cystic fibrosis, where each team member's roles are usually defined by a specific set of responsibilities, the roles of the HIV-AIDS health care team members are typically enmeshed. The parents of a child with leukemia will undoubtedly ask questions dealing with laboratory test results and disease progression. In most instances, these concerns would be addressed by a physician, and in some cases, by a nurse practitioner or clinical nurse specialist.

The social worker on the cystic fibrosis team would likely deal exclusively with concerns related to parental coping, adjustment to the diagnosis, and issues pertinent to school attendance. The HIV team social worker may deal with questions and issues related to testing and assist families in determining whether testing would be appropriate. General pediatricians, infectious disease and clinical immunology specialists may be consulted on school-related concerns in addition to medical complications.

A family affected by HIV or AIDS expects all health care team members to have a basic understanding of all aspects of HIV infection. Health care professionals should attempt to keep up to date on all new developments in the pediatric HIV and AIDS arena. The traditional lines of interdisciplinary team roles are blurred because the medical, psychosocial and legal aspects of HIV infection are not mutually exclusive. All of the medical consequences of HIV infection have psychosocial ramifications.

SOCIAL CHARACTERISTICS

To date, approximately 90% of children in the United States contracted HIV perinatally and 10% through transfusions or blood products (Personal Communication CDC, November, 1989). Until early 1987 the majority of pediatric HIV and AIDS cases in the western United States were transmitted via blood products, although at present the majority of newly diagnosed pediatric cases are transmitted perinatally. Currently, all states routinely screen donated blood for HIV antibodies. The majority of children with congenital or perinatally acquired HIV are born to mothers who have a history of intravenous (IV) drug use or whose sexual partners have displayed high risk behaviors such as IV drug use or bi-sexuality. Smaller numbers of children with HIV or AIDS contracted the virus through sexual abuse by an infected adult. Older children and adolescents who are sexually active and/or use IV drugs may be exposed by engaging in sex with an infected partner or by using a contaminated needle.

Approximately 90% of the children with AIDS are African American or Hispanic (Weinberg, Murray, 1987). The social profile of the majority of families affected by HIV-related disease clearly illustrates why coping with this condition within the context of the family unit can be devastating. The majority of families who have a child with HIV or AIDS are often female, single parent households, poor, unemployed, have a minimal educational level, substandard housing, and depend on public assistance programs for survival. HIV infection is affecting a population with minimal support and resources.

IMPLICATIONS OF DIAGNOSIS

The child at risk for HIV infection may be referred for testing and diagnostic evaluation due to a variety of factors. Many children are diagnosed because of physical symptoms and others are tested as a result of parental history. Children are also tested following the HIV or AIDS diagnosis of one or both parents.

Frequently, the families most at risk for HIV infection use the health care system in a crisis oriented, sporadic manner, and diagnosis may be delayed. When hospital emergency rooms and community clinics are utilized on a one-time basis, the physician is unable to observe a pattern of acute infections and therefore unable to make a diagnosis of HIV or AIDS. Several of the infections and complications commonly associated with childhood HIV infection include failure-to-thrive, chronic upper respiratory infections, thrush, otitis media (ear infections), malnutrition (wasting), all of which are also typical of other childhood illnesses. Other symptoms such as candida, encephalopathy, and recurrent pneumonia, are more commonly associated with HIV. Confusion in diagnosis is common, particularly if a child is not regularly seen by one physician who may also be unaware of other high risk criteria indicating a need for testing (Lewert, 1988).

A parent's preparation for the possibility of a child having AIDS begins with the time informed consent for testing is requested. Diagnosis of HIV infection in a child, regardless of the child's degree of symptomatology, results in family crisis. Equilibrium within the family system is often destroyed. Because many families at risk for HIV infection function at a limited capacity prior to the diagnosis, they may be unable to cope with the additional burden of a child with HIV.

In situations where multiple family members are infected or ill, parents are faced with the reality that they may die first and must make immediate decisions regarding alternate caretakers for their children, both those who are HIV positive and negative. When dealing with the fears surrounding disclosure of an HIV or AIDS diagnosis, one's search for an appropriate alternative caretaker is difficult. Consequently it may be in the child's best interest to be placed either with an extended family member or in the foster care system.

Following a positive test result in a child, testing for other family members may be encouraged. Although one can assume that a mother is positive, she is frequently referred for testing, either to an anonymous or confidential test site, or to a local HIV or AIDS hospital-based program. Denial is the most common defense mechanism utilized following a life-threatening diagnosis so she may not believe she is infected until she is tested. For some women, a diagnosis of HIV or AIDS may come as a complete surprise; others may be aware of risk factors in current or past behavior. It is not unusual to find that every family member has HIV or AIDS.

Other ramifications of an HIV diagnosis may include the discovery of a partner's use of IV drugs or a partner's bi-sexuality or infidelity. Decisions regarding termination of a pregnancy may also be necessary during this period.

Depression is one of the most common features in families impacted by HIV. Family member depression is compounded by fears of others' responses when told of the diagnosis of HIV or AIDS. Thus, many families find it difficult to maintain their activities of daily living when burdened by stress and anticipatory grief. In any case, coping mechanisms previously utilized to deal with other stressful life events are insufficient when the psychosocial factors of HIV infection come into play.

At the time a child is diagnosed, parents often experience varying degrees of guilt and anger. For the mother who has transmitted the virus to her child and engaged in high risk behavior, the guilt may be particularly stressful. Anger is often directed toward the partner known to have infected the woman prior to or during her pregnancy.

Although transfusion or hemophilia-related HIV is thought to be the more socially acceptable mode of transmission, and individuals are not considered to be at fault, feelings of guilt and anger still exist. Guilt may be experienced by a mother who has questions regarding her prenatal care or nutrition during her pregnancy. Anger may be directed toward individuals known to have donated blood, or toward the hospital or other health care institutions where the transfusion or clotting factor was dispensed. Regardless of the mode of transmission, parents must deal with the isolation and stigma created by this disease (Septimus, 1989).

FAMILY INTERVENTION

At the time a child is diagnosed with any chronic illness, education for the family is of paramount importance. The health care team is called upon to assist the family cope with the potentially life-threatening disease and deal with the child's changing health care and social needs. The family may need assistance to deal with the emotional impact of the illness, and the impending long-term financial hardship. All interactions with family members should be racially and culturally sensitive. Whenever possible, professionals representative of these groups should be recruited to work with families diagnosed with HIV and AIDS.

Additionally, when the child is HIV symptomatic, the family often needs assistance in managing tasks related to care of the ill child, particularly if the parent(s)' health is also deteriorating. Particular attention should be given to AIDS-related dementia in one or both parents. In these instances, collaboration with health care members caring for the parents, such as occupational therapy and psychiatry, is indicated. Ongoing communication with medical staff involved in caring for the parent(s) is important for periodic reevaluation.

Other immediate problems include issues surrounding decisions about to whom the diagnosis should be disclosed and how to anticipate and plan for their reactions. All members of the multidisciplinary team may be involved in assisting the family in these tasks. Health care providers may be biased based on personal experiences after working with many similar families; however, it is important that families be empowered to make their own decisions and choices. The role of the professional should be to outline options available, provide counselling as warranted, and assist the family in making critical decisions. Often, participation in decision making may be the family's only means of control over this devastating situation (Lewert, 1988).

During the crisis period following diagnosis, frequent discussions should take place with parents. Due to the immediate shock usually accompanying diagnosis, and the overwhelming number of topics needing to be discussed, explanations often need to be repeated several times before a family member is able to fully understand. The way the immediate crisis is handled will make the family either stronger or weaker (Boland, 1987). From the beginning, health providers can influence coping.

The shock and disbelief experienced during the crisis period may manifest itself in denial, which may last for months and may interfere with the parent(s)' ability to comply with recommendations for the child's medical followup. This may result in difficulties, particularly if the child is already symptomatic. Additionally, a mother may tend to all of the needs of her HIV infected child while needing constant encouragement and reinforcement to get medical attention for her own HIV infection.

The entire health care team must recognize the need for ongoing psychosocial support. Although various members of the team may be more involved with this, ideally a social worker is assigned to the child and family throughout the child's illness course. Early in the diagnostic process, questions related to the scope of HIV infection and resolving issues may be involved such as dealing with the child's medical bills and outside referrals. Later in the course of the disease, this individual may assist the family with issues of grief and bereavement.

All members of the health care team must be hopeful in working with HIV impacted families, an obviously difficult task in lieu of the hopeless nature of the situation. It is often through help from caregivers that families are able to remain optimistic and continue coping with the tragedies related to the diagnosis of their child. The focus of all intervention should be on the child living with AIDS, although families are well aware that HIV infection may be fatal from the start. Hope can sometimes be generated through a family's involvement in securing outside resources to help care for the child, such as day care, participation in social activities, and use of emergency support services.

Support groups have historically been used as a mode of psychosocial intervention to assist parents in coping with chronic and life-threatening diseases of children. For parents who have children with HIV infection or other chronic illnesses, groups can provide a safe, supportive environment to discuss experiences, seek advice, and alleviate some of the isolation commonly experienced. Pediatric AIDS programs across the country have reported varying degrees of success in attempting to provide ongoing support groups for these parents.

Frequently, due to the chaotic, dysfunctional nature of many families, attending a weekly or bi-weekly support group is a low priority compared to the many other priorities existing when caring for a child with a chronic illness. The daily turmoil of securing food and shelter, coupled with numerous medical appointments for various family members, is frequently more than a parent can handle. Support groups are most utilized when they take place at the time a child is seen for outpatient clinic visits. Several pediatric AIDS programs have very successfully included extended family members, caretakers and foster parents in groups.

THE CHILD WITH AIDS

A topic of growing attention has been the child who has been diagnosed with HIV infection. To date infants and children have had limited life spans but new therapeutic agents may permit these children to live longer. Thus, in recent months parents as well as health care providers working with these children have debated issues pertaining to the child's knowledge of his or her own HIV infection.

Although some parents have chosen to be open with latency age children about the name and nature of the illness, this remains a closely guarded secret in most families. Parents usually attribute their desire to keep the diagnosis a secret from the HIV infected child to one or more of the following factors: (1) disclosure to others will result in devastating consequences for the family, (2) the perception that the child will be unable to cope, (3) fear of death, (4) curiosity about how the child contracted the disease, and/or (5) parental belief that the child is better not knowing the name of his/her diagnosis.

The information a child is given must be age-appropriate — emotionally, developmentally and cognitively. This is particularly significant as these children often suffer from progressive HIV-related encephalopathy. Honest answers according to the child's age and level of understanding will help avoid future problems. Psychological intervention for the child may be appropriate, depending on the child's individual needs. Parents and other caretakers may be additionally encumbered by guilt when they most need to be honest with the child.

In some situations, particularly with older children, parents construct an alternative diagnosis which is socially acceptable, such as leukemia, in hopes that they will receive support and avoid stigma. Unfortunately, this further perpetuates the cycle of guilt. Parents can gradually get caught up in perpetuating these "half-truths."

Health care team members should incorporate the child's needs in all ongoing discussions with parents. Child development specialists can be consulted regarding the amount and detail of information given to the child. As children with HIV infection or AIDS begin to live longer, this debate with continue. Early in the diagnostic process, health care providers must pave the way for ongoing discussion with parents on this issue as the child grows older. Constant re-evaluation of the child's developmental status is critical.

The non-infected siblings of the HIV infected child, not unlike the siblings of other children with chronic disorders, are often the "forgotten group" (Brett, 1988). Stress and crisis often result in psychopathology for siblings in addition to parents. Intervention by the health care team should include advocacy on behalf of siblings to include opportunities for socialization in addition to mental health intervention. Because the non-infected child may be the only member of the nuclear family to survive, bonds with extended family members should be encouraged.

SCHOOL

The issue of school attendance by children with HIV infection has been the source of much conflict in the last few years. Although many individuals strongly object to children with HIV being mainstreamed into schools, attendance in public schools is supported by Public Law 94-142.

The primary concern is that the child will be susceptible to infection because of immune system deterioration. In some cases, home tutoring is most appropriate. In the past, attention was focused on the risk of the HIV-infected child to others within the school setting but presently this is not usually an issue. The health care team is often involved in assisting families determine whether their child needs additional assistance, sometimes related to HIV-related encephalopathy, that may not be available in a public school.

Most families whose children attend school do not disclose the diagnosis of HIV. In a questionnaire administered to parents of children with HIV and AIDS in Los Angeles, California, of 46 children attending school, both public and private, only 6 families had disclosed the diagnosis. The 6 who had disclosed did so for at least one of the following reasons: (1) frequent absences, (2) medication needs during the school day, (3) fear of exposure to routine infections (physician advised disclosure), and/or (4) HIV encephalopathy, causing developmental delay and a resulting need for special classes. Many public school districts across the country have developed policies for the confidential mainstreaming of children from kindergarten through the twelfth grade.

OUTSIDE RESOURCES

In the process of developing a multidisciplinary treatment plan for the family, the use of community resources is often essential. Clearly, many agencies and services utilized by the family prior to the diagnosis of HIV may be unwilling to provide services once the diagnosis is known. Families are most comfortable when support services personnel are aware of the child's illness and are able to provide supportive and compassionate care.

Various team members may be called upon to provide education to service providers to help them overcome their fears and to determine their capability to provide the type of care needed. Although many community agencies that provide services to adults with AIDS may be capable of meeting some of the needs of the pediatric population, families usually feel most comfortable utilizing services historically geared toward the needs of chronically ill children and their families. Each family should be reviewed regularly to insure that needs are adequately met, and not perceived as being insignificant when the family has difficulty obtaining services.

THE HEALTH CARE WORKER

The complex psychosocial issues of childhood HIV and AIDS, combined with multiple family difficulties, present unique challenges to health care professionals. For the most part, the already chaotic families become increasingly dysfunctional as the medical status of family members deteriorates. Family members frequently miss scheduled appointments with medical and ancillary services. Concrete needs such as utilities and housing are paramount. Contacts tend to be crisis oriented and do not allow time to address educational and supportive issues.

The health care professionals who work with these families are constantly under stress. Many feelings of frustration arise because families with HIV or AIDS are difficult to reach, and it is difficult to have a positive impact. Social workers may feel that further intervention to assist parents in coping with the illness of their child is prohibited because so much time is spent on the concrete needs of these families. Hospitals and community agencies should be encouraged to take an active role in the education and support of health care providers. Employee support networks can provide nurses and other health professionals with an opportunity to ventilate their feelings of stress and anxiety and hopefully prevent "burn out." This will be even more essential as the numbers of children with HIV and AIDS increase.

CONCLUSION

This review has presented the myriad of psychosocial issues for families who have a child who has been diagnosed with HIV infection. Health care workers often have the most significant role in supporting a family in their attempts to cope with the day-to-day challenges of having a child with a devastating illness. As we embark into the second decade of perhaps the greatest public health challenge of all time, we must constantly consider the unique psychosocial problems that further delineate this disease from any other affecting mankind.

STUDY QUESTIONS

1. *Delineate the psychosocial factors that set HIV/AIDS apart from other childhood chronic illnesses.*
2. *Specify issues that families need to consider when making school related decisions.*

3. *Describe the importance of health care providers understanding the psychosocial ramifications of pediatric HIV infection.*

REFERENCES

Boland, M.G., (1987). The child with AIDS special concern. In T.S. Durham & F.L. Cohen (Eds.), *The person with AIDS: Nursing perspective* (pp. 192-210), New York: Springer.

Brett, K.M., (1988). Sibling response to chronic childhood disorders: Research perspectives and practice implications. *Issues in Comprehensive Pediatric Nursing, 11,* 43-57.

Koop, C.E., (1987, April 6-8). Excerpts from Keynote Address. In Report of Surgeon General's Workshop on Children with HIV Infection and Their Families. U.S. Department of Health and Human Services, 3-5.

Lewert, G., (1988, June). Children and AIDS. *Journal of Contemporary Social Work,* 348-351.

Nelson, L.P., (1987, September-October). AIDS: children with HIV infection and their families. *Journal of Dentistry for Children,* 353-358.

Septimus, A., (1989, February). Psycho-social aspects of caring for families of infants infected with human immunodeficiency virus. *Seminars in Perinatology,* 39-54.

Weinberg, D.S. & Murray, H.W., (1987). Coping with AIDS: The special problems of New York City. *New England Journal of Medicine, 317(23),* 1469-1473.

Women and AIDS:
Implications for Occupational Therapists

Wendy Wood, MA, OTR/L
Mary Ruth Aull, BSN, RN

SUMMARY. This article examines the special issues which confront women with AIDS. The population of women with AIDS is described and differences in the course of the disease between women and men are briefly explored. The pyschosocial responses of women with AIDS are reviewed with respect to considerations of stigma, informational needs, economic impact, psychological responses and social supports. Lastly, the role of occupational therapy is described as it relates to enabling and empowering women with AIDS to perform daily activities and role obligations and to achieve terminal occupational goals.

INTRODUCTION

The rate of increase in women [with AIDS] is alarming. Between January and September, 1988, the proportion of AIDS cases occurring in women was 10 percent; prior to 1988, the proportion was about 7 percent. It is estimated that between 1 million and 1.5 million Americans are now infected with HIV [human immunodeficiency virus]; approximately 100,000 of these are thought to be women of child bearing age. . . . (Public Health Reports, 1988, p. 88)

It would be difficult to dispute the notion that the AIDS pandemic has provided the definitive diagnostic test of the deficiencies of our current health care system. Without doubt, the complex issues facing women with

Wendy Wood is Clinical Supervisor in the Occupational Therapy Department at Harmarville Rehabilitation Center in Pittsburgh, PA.
Mary Ruth Aull is Research Nurse Specialist with the AIDS Trial Group of the Graduate School of Public Health, University of Pittsburgh.

AIDS has sharpened the diagnostic power of this disease. When AIDS was viewed as a disease limited primarily to gay or bisexual men and intravenous (IV) drug abusers, health care providers were confronted with the need to examine their values and reactions to certain high risk "groups."

The growing number of women with AIDS, on the other hand, represents an ethnically and socially diverse population which is inclusive of the white, heterosexual "mainstream." At the same time, however, and perhaps paradoxically, women with AIDS, when viewed as a group, point out the profound impact of race, class, and economic inequalities upon health and illness. While their experience parallels those of men in many respects, women living with AIDS raise additional issues concerning access to health care, as well as lifelong access to societal institutions designed to impart both hope and skill for the future.

The purpose of this article is to provide an overview of the special issues which confront women with AIDS and secondly, to describe the role of occupational therapy with this population. Topics covered include epidemiologic characteristics of women with AIDS, the transmission of HIV to women, the medical course of AIDS in women, and psychosocial responses of women with AIDS. It is proposed that by applying a generalist's perspective, occupational therapists may assist women with AIDS in accomplishing required and chosen daily activities as well as terminal occupational goals.

BACKGROUND

Who are the women with AIDS? An epidemiological study between the years of 1981 to 1986 indicated that, of the total population of women with AIDS, 52% were IV drug users, 21% were sexual partners of men at risk for AIDS, 10% were recipients of blood transfusions, 1% had hemophilia or a coagulation disorder, and 11% had undetermined risk factors (Guinan & Hardy, 1986). A disproportionately high percentage of women with AIDS are women of color. In the United States, while Afro Americans comprise 12% of the total population and Hispanics 6%, 50% of women with AIDS are Afro American and 22% are Hispanic (Kawata & Gerald, 1987). Of all pediatric AIDS cases, a full 80% are minority infants and children (Kawata & Gerald, 1987). Quite significantly, the large majority of women with AIDS (79%) are within their childbearing years, ranging in age from 13 to 39 years of age (Wofsy, 1987).

In human terms, these are snapshots of women behind the statistics:

A mother and grandmother whose gay son died of AIDS five years ago. Her partner died last year of AIDS. Despite her losses, she states that this past year is the best year of her life. She has become a spokeswoman and role model for women with AIDS.

A woman with AIDS [who] shared needles with her husband, yet did not know of the risk in 1981. Three of her children died from AIDS in infancy. She and her husband also died. She is remembered fondly for her humor and her strength. . . .

A woman with AIDS who has a female partner with children. They shared needles and were prostitutes. They are a family, yet were denied access to family shelters because they are a lesbian couple. They chose to live together on the streets as a family.

A woman with AIDS who had one sex partner five years after her divorce. She was unaware that he was in a high-risk group. Unable to afford adequate housing, she lives with a large extended family. Everyone in the family tells her not to worry or cry. Her teenage son withdraws into silence.

A woman with AIDS whose husband was an IV drug user. She returned to care for him when he was dying although he had beaten her. She simply says, "There was no one else to do it. . . ."

A woman with AIDS who stole to feed her children. At work she listens in silence to coworkers' AIDS jokes. She fears losing her job and her children. (Maier, 1986, p. 5-6)

As illustrated by these brief portrayals, the reality of women with AIDS cannot be reduced to the purely medical aspects of their illness. In 1983, the Public Health Service Task Force on Women's Health Issues identified the following factors as relating significantly to the health of women: "cultural/social values and attitudes; economic status; labor force participation; family, household structure, and social support systems; and, interactions with the health care system" (Public Health Reports, 1988, p. 88). These factors may negatively affect a woman living with AIDS as well as a woman's risk of becoming HIV infected.

Similarly, the day to day reality of women living with AIDS is inseparable from a myriad of occupational roles such as worker, mother, family provider, spouse, or health care provider to children and partners with AIDS (Public Health Reports, 1988). Many women with AIDS simultaneously suffer from addictions and are from the most economically and educationally disadvantaged segment of our society. In short, to understand a woman with AIDS, one must understand the developmental, social, economic and cultural matrix of her life.

TRANSMISSION OF HIV TO WOMEN

HIV has been isolated from peripheral blood cells, cerebral spinal fluid, brain tissue, urine, saliva, semen, tears, and vaginal and cervical fluids or cells (Wofsy et al., 1986). Direct exposure to any of these body fluids, even if contaminated with HIV, does not necessarily present a risk for infection. The risk of transmission appears to be dependent upon both the type of the body fluid which is encountered and the anatomic area which is exposed (Peterman & Curran, 1986). Blood, semen, and vaginal secretions have considerably higher concentrations of HIV than do tears and saliva. This is because the virus prefers lymphocytes (Peterman & Curran, 1986). The virus is not believed to cross intact skin, but rather to enter an uninfected individual through disruptions of the mucous membranes (Peterman & Curran, 1986).

IV drug users who shared needles with HIV positive individuals face the highest risk of infection as a result of direct intravenous contact with infected blood. IV drug users constitute the greatest proportion of women with AIDS. These women have historically been isolated from mainstream institutions. Often they have had considerable difficulty interacting with the health care system and receiving adequate care.

Heterosexual intercourse with a partner at risk for AIDS is the second most common mode of transmission of HIV infection to women (Guinan & Hardy, 1986). As there are a greater number of men with AIDS, women are more likely than men to encounter an infected partner. Additionally, the transmission of HIV from man to woman may be more efficient than from woman to man (Guinan & Hardy, 1986). Heterosexual women are thus at greater risk for HIV infection through sexual intercourse than are heterosexual men (Guinan & Hardy, 1987).

Heterosexual contact is the only transmission category where numbers of women with AIDS is greater than the number of men with AIDS. According to Guinan and Hardy (1987), "the proportion of women with AIDS in the heterosexual contact category increased from 12% to 16% between 1982 and 1986" (p. 2040). In their study of women who had acquired AIDS through heterosexual contact, 67% of the women's sexual partners were IV drug users, 16% were bisexual men, 1% were men with hemophilia, and 16% were men with undetermined risk factors.

Women have also acquired HIV through artificial insemination of infected semen into the uterus through a catheter (Stewart et al., 1985).

When skin or mucous membrane are not intact, direct transmission of the virus into the blood can occur during artificial insemination. The risk of exposure through artificial insemination may be significantly reduced through screening of donors for HIV exposure, cryopreservation of semen for a minimum of three months, and retesting of donors for HIV infection before use of semen (Stewart et al., 1985).

Given that a high frequency of sexual contacts is associated with HIV infection (Padian et al., 1987), prostitution increases the risk for HIV infection and thus to its transmission ("Antibody," 1987). There has not been adequate scientific evidence, however, to confirm that female prostitutes are a major source of transmission of HIV to heterosexual men (Anderson, 1987). Consistent with the predominant transmission category for women in general, IV drug abuse has been identified as the major risk factor for HIV infection in prostitutes ("Antibody," 1987).

THE MEDICAL COURSE OF AIDS IN WOMEN

HIV infected women differ from men in symptomatology and are often diagnosed at a later stage in the disease than men (Maier, 1986). Since the diagnosis of women generally occurs later than it does for men, women are often sicker when finally treated. Chronic vaginitis has been reported to be a common presenting complaint. Kaposi's sarcoma or involvement of the central nervous system is somewhat less prevalent in women with AIDS or AIDS Related Complex (ARC) than with men.

It appears that women also die sooner of the disease than do men (Klosser, 1988). Because of this, health care providers working with women need to be aware of early signs of HIV infection and need to know when to refer for HIV testing. Similarly, it is of vital importance that community-based health care and physical, emotional, and spiritual support be made available to women who test HIV positive or who manifest the early stages of AIDS or ARC.

PSYCHOSOCIAL RESPONSES OF WOMEN WITH AIDS

Macks (1986) identified five areas which highlight significant psychosocial responses of people with AIDS and ARC. These include *stigma, informational needs, economic impact/concrete needs, psychological and emotional responses*, and *social supports*. While applicable to both men and women, women present with special concerns in each of these areas.

Stigma

Because the AIDS epidemic has been associated with risk behaviors of homosexuality and drug use, persons with AIDS are socially stigmatized. Women, regardless of how they became HIV infected, do not escape the effects of social stigma (Macks, 1986). According to Maier (1986), "These women are assumed to be prostitutes, or to be promiscuous. . . . These women feel shame, fear, and guilt" (p. 1-2).

Women not only must deal with the stigma associated with their partner, they may become targets of blame for having transmitted AIDS to their children (Macks, 1986). Given the role of women in society, women additionally contend with discrimination resulting from the devaluation of their gender (Mack, 1986). The effects of stigma, blame, and discrimination upon women are to underscore feelings of personal guilt and shame and to heigahten isolation from social and medical supports.

Informational Needs

Due to the diversity of women with AIDS, specific informational needs are apparent with respect to prevention of HIV infection and management of the disease. Prevention information must be culturally and socially sensitized to Afro American and Hispanic women. In addition, prevention information must be specifically targeted to reach women who are IV drug abusers as well as non-addicted heterosexual women who may believe that they are not at risk for HIV infection. Women with AIDS require basic medical information concerning opportunistic infections, neurological complications, management of dementia, and dietary needs. Information is also necessary regarding the special needs of infants and children with HIV infection and methods of access to health care, housing and child care.

Economic Impact

As a group, women are more economically disadvantaged than men. Accordingly, the economic impact of AIDS upon women, whether they have children or not, is often quite profound. Women with children may have difficulty finding affordable housing in areas which are safe for both themselves and their children. As a result, they may be forced to give up custody in order to acquire safe and adequate housing for both themselves and their children (Maier, 1986).

Women who maintain custody are often the sole economic providers for their children. Child care is an especially important service for these women. According to Macks (1986), "women with children need child care services not only for the times they are too ill to care for their children, but for the time consuming task of dealing with a life threatening illness" (p. 7). Child care services and family support services may be extremely marginal or altogether lacking in economically deprived areas where many women with AIDS live.

Psychological Responses

The psychological responses of women with AIDS are similar to those of persons diagnosed with terminal illnesses. At the same time, these responses must be understood within the context of the specter of AIDS itself, that is, the stigmatizing aspect of the disease and its specific interpersonal, economic, social, and cultural dimensions. Grief reactions approximate those of patients diagnosed with cancer with potential progression through the stages of denial, anger, bargaining, depression, and acceptance (Macks, 1986). As physical and cognitive states fluctuate and progressively deteriorate, the person with AIDS often experiences an emotional roller coaster characterized by crisis and adaptation to crisis.

In addition to managing the medical aspects of the disease, women with AIDS must manage feelings of despair and hopelessness, often exacerbated by the prevalence of the disease or HIV infection in their children and significant others. Loss of the ability to function in maternal or caregiving roles may be particularly distressing. According to Macks (1986), "many women with HIV have been mothers and caretakers their entire lives, relying on these roles as their source of self-esteem. As they get sicker, their ability to maintain these roles diminishes, precipitating a distressing identity crisis" (p.11-12). Many women must confront and plan for the reality of leaving their children motherless and potentially homeless when they die. Denial, continued substance abuse, and/or isolation from support services may be particularly problematic issues.

Spiritual beliefs and maintaining hope have been found to be positively associated with the ability to live effectively with AIDS (Macks, 1986). Taking action such as making desired life changes, starting a relationship, exerting control over medical decisions, becoming politically active, or developing a spiritual practice has helped many people with AIDS to maintain a sense of hope (Macks. 1986). Support groups have been found to be effective in helping women to mobilize and achieve personal, family, and political goals (Maier, 1986).

Social Support

Women with AIDS are at high risk for having their intimate sexual relationships and family systems deteriorate and eventually break apart. Intimacy and sexuality are profoundly affected as women with AIDS often "feel sexually dirty and unloved. They believe they have lost the American image of femininity and withdraw further because of their appearance" (Maier, 1986, p. 4). Of thirty-two women in one support group, only three had relationships that remained intact after they were diagnosed with AIDS or ARC (Maier, 1986).

Family systems risk fracture due to lack of economic and social support in addition to the effects of addictive disease upon familial relationships and stability (Macks, 1986). Yet, AIDS resources do not generally incorporate a family model (Maier, 1986). Because HIV infection initially appeared to be unique to the gay and bisexual male population, most community supports are presently geared for males. Fewer support services are available to heterosexual couples or to women with children. In contrast to many gay and bisexual men with AIDS, most women with AIDS do not have the support of a politically active and emotionally supportive community.

OCCUPATIONAL THERAPY AND WOMEN WITH AIDS

Occupational therapy for women with AIDS presents great challenges and equally great rewards. If one is to be an effective occupational therapist with this population, a generalist's perspective is necessary. More importantly, however, occupational therapists must base their interventions upon an understanding of the co-existing physical, mental, affective and spiritual experiences of women living with AIDS, as well as the interpersonal, social, and cultural dimensions of this disease. Intervention hinges upon the belief that women with AIDS can be empowered to take control of their lives by making choices for effective occupational behavior.

At the physical and mental levels of occupational functioning, occupational therapists assist women with AIDS through clinical interventions most commonly associated with physical disabilities and psychosocial specialty areas of practice. Specifically, techniques of environmental adaptation, energy conservation, work simplification, and activity analysis and adaptation are applied to enabling performance of required and chosen activities of daily living. To maintain optimal physical capability, self-care often focuses upon maintenance of adequate nutrition and effective habits in planning and preparing food.

With respect to the affective, volitional, and spiritual dimensions of women with AIDS, occupational therapist address a plethora of concerns. These include the meaningfulness, self-esteem, and value associated with specific occupations and occupational roles, choices regarding time use, self-efficacy with respect to achieving goals in the face of a terminal and progressive illness, and beliefs concerning hope for the future and the importance of planning for life goals. Specific interventions may focus upon developing skill in the maternal role, adapting the maternal role when the mother has beginning dementia, or adapting the worker role to allow continued participation. Individual and group activities may be used therapeutically to enhance effective time use as well as to assist in identifying and pursuing terminal occupational goals.

Occupational therapy must be inclusive of the family systems of women with AIDS in order to be optimally effective and relevant. In addition, occupational therapists should be sensitized to, and respectful of, the cultural backgrounds of women with AIDS. As with treating men with AIDS, occupational therapists must be supportive of the need for interdisciplinary interventions which address the complexity of the medical, psychosocial, and spiritual experiences of living with AIDS. Lastly, occupational therapists must themselves believe that AIDS can be transformed from inevitable personal tragedy to triumph of the human spirit. As summarized by Maier (1986):

> These women are indeed a diverse group with many specific needs and concerns. They are isolated and devastated by this disease, yet they seem to emerge. They develop new strength and power they did not have before. They speak at conferences and to other people with AIDS. They bond with and support women, some for the first time in their male-oriented lives. They express that they feel like real people. They learn to say no. They support and nurture the community of men with AIDS and accept that nurturing can be good for them. They are moving toward becoming whole people. They are taking their power and are organizing . . . to develop their own resources and to risk discrimination by speaking to the media and the general public. They are beginning to feel less isolated and that they matter. (p. 4-5)

REFERENCES

Anderson, P., (1987). *Summary of data on prostitutes and AIDS*. National Task Force on Prostitution.

Antibody to human immunodeficiency virus in female prostitutes, (1987). *Journal of the American Medical Association*, 257, 2011-2012.

Guinan, M. and Hardy, A., (1987). Epidemiology of AIDS in women in the United States. *Journal of the American Medical Association*, 257, 2039-2042.

Kawata, P. and Gerald, G., (1987). *AIDS education and support services to minorities: A survey of community based AIDS service providers*. Washington, DC: National AIDS Network.

Klosser, P., (1988). A doctor tells women they are at risk. *AIDS Patient Care*, 2, 3-4.

Macks, J., (1986). Psychosocial responses of people with AIDS/ARC. (Women and AIDS: Clinical Resource Guide). San Francisco, CA: San Francisco AIDS Foundation.

Maier, C., (1986). Women with AIDS and ARC in San Francisco. (Woman and AIDS: Clinical Resource Guide). San Francisco, CA: San Francisco AIDS Foundation.

Padian, N., Marquis, L., Francis, D., Anderson, R., Rutherford, G., O'Malley, P., Winkelstein, W., (1987). Male-to-female transmission of human immunodeficiency virus. *Journal of the American Medical Association*, 258, 788-790.

Peterman, T. and Curran, J., (1986). Sexual transmission of human immunodeficiency virus. *Journal of the American Medical Association*, 256, 2222-2225.

Public Health Reports, (1988). *Cross-Cutting Issues: Women and AIDS* (Supp. No. 1-89), *103*, 88-98.

Stewart, G., Tyler, J., Cunningham, A., Barr, J., Driscoll, G., Gold, J., Lamont, B., (1985). Transmission of human T-cell lymphotropic virus Type III (HTLV-III) by artificial insemination by donor. *The Lancet, September*, 581-584.

Wofsy, C., (1987). Human immunodeficiency virus infection in women. *Journal of the American Medical Association*, 257, 2074-2076.

Wofsy, C., Cohen, J., Hauer, L., Padian, N., Michaelis, B., Evans, L., Levy, J., (1986). Isolation of AIDS-Associated retrovirus from genital secretions of women with antibodies to the virus. *The Lancet, March*, 527-529.

Pain Management
and Neuromuscular Reeducation
for the HIV Patient

Mary Lou Galantino, MS, PT

SUMMARY. As a multisystem chronic illness, two areas come to the forefront for management by the rehabilitation specialist. Pain and neuromuscular deficits may be a result of direct insult by the human immunodeficiency virus (HIV) or opportunistic infections affecting functional abilities. A brief overview of pathologic findings reveals that the types of pain experiences is based upon the disease processes that are occurring secondary to HIV. The management of pain and resultant functional changes depends on the source, symptoms and signs of pain. Physical and Occupational therapists are key health care professionals to conduct pain assessments and evaluate functional impairment to better employ non-invasive techniques for management of HIV complications. This article presents various modalities and modes of therapeutic intervention to enhance full participation of the person with HIV in activities of daily living.

INTRODUCTION

The progression of HIV infection displays a number of pathological changes. As therapists, we often focus on the projected linear progress of our patients. However, with HIV patients, we find a vascillation of progress and regression that forces us away from our traditional methods of

Mary Lou Galantino has devoted her career to HIV clinical research. She has published numerous articles on rehabilitation and HIV infection. She has presented at national and international conferences on cancer, AIDS and chronic pain. Former Director of Physical Therapy at the Institute for Immunological Disorders in Houston, TX, Mary Lou is now the owner of LIFE Physical Therapy, a private practice in Houston. She is also Contributing Editor/Consultant for the Physical Therapy Forum.

161

practice. This population is remarkable in that it exhibits dramatic swings in the time frame and severity of relapses. Commonly seen physical manifestations of illness are neuromusular disorders and pain. Physical and Occupational Therapists are in an optimal position to perform pain and strength assessments and provide interventions to improve overall functional abilities in the HIV patient.

This article will review pain syndromes most commonly seen in patients with HIV and discuss changes in neuromuscular status. Strategies for intervention, including manual therapy techniques, will also be described.

PAIN SYNDROMES

Although there has been a dramatic increase in the number of patients with AIDS, there is a lack of literature about the prevalence of pain or descriptions of different pain syndromes in these patients. The symptom of pain may be overshadowed by a constellation of other overwhelming problems, which may include opportunistic infections, dyspnea, anorexia, and neuropsychological symptoms found in many HIV patients.

Postural changes secondary to rapid muscle wasting may create trigger points and associated referred pain. Dermatological manifestations of herpes zoster are painful and may persist long after open lesions subside. Side effects from chemotherapeutic agents include peripheral neuropathies, predominantly a distal symmetrical sensory neuropathy with painful paresthesias being the main clinical problem (Galantino, 1987). Peripheral neuropathies may be manifesed as causalgia, which produces a burning sensation and trophic skin changes, causing highly sensitive trigger point areas. Paresthesia is another pain sensation associated with this and may be perceived as an electrical sensation along the course of the nerve root. The patient may be extremely hypersensitive and guarded about touch because it might exacerbate the perception of pain.

The possible causes of most of the pain syndromes or sites are complex. The highest incidence of chest pain was presumed to be secondary to the prevalence of pneumocystic carinii pneumonia (PCP). The etiology of the pain must be delineated for appropriate therapeutic intervention. With the advent of successful drug interventions, rehabilitation specialists observe a wide range of physiological deficits, resulting in an altered functional status. Neurological disorders may also complicate all stages of HIV infection, and some degenerative disorders may cause pain (Galantino and Levy, January, 1988). Common causes of headache are toxoplasmosis, cryptococcus meningitis, central nervous system lymphoma and nonspecific lymphoma.

NEUROMUSCULAR COMPLICATIONS

The musculoskeletal system is often compromised secondary to HIV infection. Muscle weakness associated with malignancies includes polymyopathy, polymyositis, disorders of neuromuscular function, metabolic myopathies and myopathies secondary to disordered endocrine secretion (Galantino, 1987). In most cases, the etiology of direct or indirect effects of paraneoplastic progress on muscle function is unknown. This is also true for the patient with HIV. Simpson, Bender and Herman (1986) reported cases of polymyositis in AIDS patients. Serum CPK was markedly elevated and EMG indicated denervation and myopathy. Muscle biopsy revealed inflammatory myopathy, and electron miscroscopic studies found retrovirus-type particles. Cryptococcus and toxoplasma myopathy have also been reported to demonstrate the effects of opportunistic infections in various pain syndromes and muscular deficits throughout the course of HIV.

TREATMENT APPROACHES

Modalities

A multi-modality approach, including transcutaneous electric nerve stimulation (TENS), microamperage current, a pain supressor and manual therapy techniques, is a consideration for treatment of these pain syndromes (Galantino and Brewer, 1989). An important aspect of pain management is focusing on posture and body awareness. This emphasis on the body and its alignment may reduce pain associated with the rapid musculoskeletal change observed in many patients. Body image as perceived by the patient should be enhanced throughout the rehabilitation process to allow expression of the rapid changes that can occur.

Manual Therapy

Manual therapy techniques are beneficial adjuvants particularly when the virus has invaded the central or peripheral nervous systems or when opportunistic infections have caused viral related myelitis. Myofascial release and craniosacral therapy are specific techniques for HIV patients to relieve pain and restore function. These techniques are non-invasive, gentle and an effective addition to the therapists' repertoire of techniques.

The importance of the role of the fascial system in pain and dysfunction has been documented by Upledger and Vredevoogd (1983). Malfunction, or the binding down of the fascia, may be the reason for various pain syndromes. The fascia is a tough connective tissue which spreads three dimensionally throughout the body without interruption. The fascia surrounds all of the somatic and visceral structures of the human body. Therefore, malfunction of the fascial system due to trauma, posture or inflammation can create a binding down of the fascia, resulting on abnormal pressure on nerves, muscles, bones or organs. This can create pain or malfunction, sometimes with side effects and seemingly unrelated symptoms not always following a specific pain pattern (Barnes, August, 1984). It is difficult to diagnose because the standard tests that an HIV patient may undergo to determine the etiology of pain (CT, myelograms, X-rays) do not demonstrate the fascia.

The fascia can be delineated by (1) superficial fascia, which lies directly below the dermis; (2) deep fascia, which surrounds and infuses with muscle, bone, nerves, blood vessels and organs of the body at the cellular level; and (3) deepest fascia, which is in the dura of the cranial sacral system. A whole body phenomenon is represented when one considers that these are arbitrary divisions. The superficial fascia affects the deep fascia, and the deep fascia affects the fascia within the craniosacral system. The opposite is also true, creating an open system within the human body, where each fascial level affects the others. Fascia at the cellular level create the interstitial spaces and have extremely important functions in support, protection, separation, cellular respiration, elimination, metabolism, and fluid and lymphatic flow. Given that all of these systems are affected in the HIV patient, any trauma or malfunction of the fascia can set up the body's environment for poor cellular efficiency, pain and dysfunction.

The craniosacral concept is a potent therapeutic vision grounded upon certain anatomical, physiological and therapeutic observations. The cranial sacral system has a rhythmic, mobile activity which persists throughout life with normal rhythm ranging between 6 to 12 cycles per minute. In non-pathological circumstances, the rate of craniosacral rhythmic motion is quite stable. It does not fluctuate as do the rates of the cardiovascular and respiratory systems in response to exercise, motion and rest. Therefore it is reliable criterion for the evaluation of pathological conditions. It has been observed that patients suffering from acute illnesses with fever will exhibit abnormally rapid rates (Upledger and Vredevoogd, 1983). Incorporating craniosacral and myofascial techniques are particularly effective throughout the spectrum of HIV diseases, as the patient experiences multiple episodes of fever secondary to opportunistic infections.

The neuromuscular insults to the HIV infected individual as the disease progresses lead to a myriad of problems. These can range from central nervous system infections, vascular complications, spinal cord dysfunction, neoplasms and myopathies (American Association of Immunologists, 1989). The craniosacral system is clearly disrupted by neuromuscular insults. Craniosacral therapy techniques can be incorporated in a pain management program to relieve pain, restore function and empower individuals to live productively.

Although it has been taught that the cranial bones do not move, it has been documented in over three hundred studies that the cranial bones do move via the mechanism of the cerebral spinal fluid (CSF) (Upledger and Vredevoogd, 1983). CSF production in the choroid plexus of the ventricles of the brain increases the pressure within this semi-enclosed hydraulic system. The arachnoid granulation body, which is a sinusoidal plexus of blood vessels that becomes engorged, acts like a ball valve mechanism in the straight sinus. This blocks the great cerebral vein and increases the pressure within the cranial vault. This gaps the cranial suture which is under hemostatic control. At a certain point, as the suture spreads, a signal is sent to the brain to cease the production of cerebral spinal fluid. When the cranial sutures compress again, the intersutural material becomes compressed and sends a message to the brain to resume production of the CSF. This has an effect not only on the cranium, but throughout the body. Given the multiple insults to the central and peripheral nervous systems in the HIV patient, a direct alteration in the cranial system is apparent. If there is a binding down of the fascia anywhere in the body (due to local inflammation or lymphadenopathy), there can be profound and deleterious effects throughout the body. These can affect one's health and sense of well being and can create pain and dysfunction.

As one performs this therapy, pathways of motion may change. It is the role of the therapist to allow the structure to move along any new pathway it desires and not allow it to return to the pathway of origin. The techniques used in craniosacral therapy are usually non-intrusive and are both indirect and direct. An indirect technique releases a restriction of abnormal barrier to motion by encouraging motion in the direction of ease. A direct technique first involves identifying a barrier to normal physiological motion. The therapist then gently assists the restricted structure or membrane to pass through and break the abnormal restriction.

The beneficial effects of many of these therapeutic techniques includes (1) fascial continuity; (2) restoration of autonomic flexibility and; (3) enhancement of the lymphatic pump (Upledger and Vredevoogd, 1983). Fascial continuity indicates that the human body fascia is continuous from the top of the head to the bottom of the feet. It is oriented in a longitudinal direction and is free to glide on the order of millimeters when the body musculature is relaxed. Autonomic flexibility is used to describe an improvement in the ability of the autonomic nervous system to respond to stress and challenge. The rationale for the use of the lymphatic pump technique is to enhance the removal of toxic waste substances from the body and to improve circulation of antibodies.

Cognitive Distraction

Anxiety related stress may be another source of pain or contribute to the existing fatigue experienced by the person with HIV. It should be recognized that the patient's physical complaints are real even though they may be secondary to emotional stress. Cognitive distraction involves a variety of techniques that manipulate the cognitive components of pain perception. The patient's stress and pain may be managed via biofeedback, creative visualization and mental imagery. By diverting attention and concentration away from pain, a combination of chemical, physiological and neuroendocrinological events establish a sense of balance. A new area of science called psychoneuroimmunology has begun to explore the chemical links between the mind and health.

Neuromuscular Reeducation

Physical characteristics of atrophy are manifested through equilibrium and coordination disturbances, ataxia and other gait problems and an overall altered functional status. Generally, primary treatment of most of the musculoskeletal and nervous system disorders associated with HIV can incorporate various techniques of neuromotor retraining. Neuromotor retraining can include proprioceptive neuromuscular facilitation (PNF), Bobath, Brunnstrom and Rood techniques.

Neuromuscular reeducation emphasizes a "hands-on" approach to treatment, and encourages full partnership of the patient. Through reeducation, the body relearns normal patterns of movement. Through this process, improvements are noted in balance and coordination, gait and transfers, activities of daily living (ADL) (e.g., bathing, dressing, grooming, eating) and in all aspects of daily functioning. People with HIV are then empowered to more independently carry out routine tasks.

Exercise Intervention

Physical activity is a spontaneous response to stress that may be considered to be effective in the management of generalized fatigue often experienced by HIV patients. Without physical activity, stress may manifest itself as chronic pain. Thus, it is advised that patients regularly engage in a variety of non-sedentary activities (Galantino and Spence, May, 1987). Since the immune, nervous and endocrine systems are intimately related, chronic anxiety may not only affect the nervous system but may suppress the immune response.

Certain measurable physiological conditions have been correlated with various degenerative diseases that are prevalent in society. In a study done by Spence, Galantino, Mossberg and Zimmerman (in press), patients who participated in a six week exercise program on the total power hydrafitness machine three times a week demonstrated significant muscle function. In the thigh muscle group, strength increased by 23%, power by 43% and endurance by 41%; chest and arm muscle groups showed a 16% increase in strength, 30% in power and 26% in endurance; in the shoulder and arm muscle groups, strength increased by 10%, power by 38% and endurance by 24%.

The results of the study indicate that muscle function of the experimental group significantly improved, whereas the control group did not. In fact, the control group lost an average of greater than 7% muscle function. Likewise, there was a significant increase in the dimensions of the major muscle exercised in the experimental group, in contrast to a loss of size in the control group. The magnitude of loss of the control group is significant when considering function needed to carry out daily living tasks.

Nutritional Considerations

A team approach is vital to successful rehabilitation of the HIV individual. The therapist, in collaboration with the nutritionist, can develop strategies to (1) meet the needs of a sound nutritional program in concert with activity level; (2) enhance fatigue tolerance, and (3) emphasize the importance of a wellness program.

The requirements for proper energy balance ideally should be based on metabolic determination rather than on empirical equations that only estimate daily energy expenditure (Garcia, Collins and Mansell, 1987). Energy metabolism should be measured under a variety of conditions including rest and both sedentary and nonsedentary activity. This is important in the development of a physical exercise program.

Endurance Retraining

Structured physical activity for the patient with HIV is appropriate in order to improve functional capacity and fatigue tolerance. Based on the patient's tolerance to exercise, the therapist should consider intensity, duration, and frequency of exercise (Lea and Febiger, 1980). Cardiovascular endurance is the primary goal of exercise therapy designed to improve functional capacity. A delicate balance between activity level and energy conservation techniques further stresses the rehabilitation team approach.

Prevention strategies in the early stages of this disease appear to be beneficial in maintaining good posture, strength and endurance. Carefully monitored programs are needed when opportunistic infections complicate the disease process. Therefore, it is a challenge to the therapist to monitor the progression of the disease in each patient and to reevaluate and adjust treatment regimens as needed.

Psychological Intervention

Psychological support is a dynamic process of HIV intervention. A study by Rigsby, Raven, Jackson, Dishman and Berk (1989) measured the effects of exercise and counseling on the physiological, psychological and immunological factors in HIV+ individuals. Both the exercise and counseling groups showed a significant decrease in depression over the treatment period. The exercise group had a positive upward trend of immunological markers (T4/T8), suggesting that an exercise program for HIV+ people can be very beneficial in improving the physiological status of these individuals while not harming their already compromised immune status.

CONCLUSION

As the HIV epidemic unfolds, the profound implications of HIV infection for the practice of rehabilitation are becoming appreciated. As therapists, we have an opportunity to effect a change in this patient population through a familiar body of knowledge. The importance of pain management and therapeutic exercise intervention can enhance the potential of individuals with HIV to engage more fully in life. Physical and occupational therapists are in an optimal position to conduct assessments to address these specific needs. We must expand beyond this to embrace the existing potential of each human being affected by HIV.

STUDY QUESTIONS

1. Discuss the several types of physical pain experienced by people with HIV infection and AIDS. Describe three treatment strategies that alleviates pain.
2. Design a physical treatment program for a person with HIV related peripheral lower extremity neuropathy and upper extremity muscle wasting. How might this program be carried out in the patient's daily schedule? How might you incorporate the caregiver who has beginning upper and lower extremity neuropathy himself?
3. Discuss how craniosacral work can assist in pain reduction and how it can complement other neuromuscular rehabilitation strategies. How might occupational and physical therapists incorporate this strategy in their work?

REFERENCES

Barnes, J.F., (1984, August). Benefits of myofascial release. *Physical Therapy Forum (Middle Atlantic Edition)*, *3*(35), 3-6.

Galantino, M.L., (1987). Overview of the AIDS patient. *Clinical Management in Physical Therapy*, *7*, 12-13.

Galantino, M.L. and Levy, J., (1988, January). HIV infection: Neurological implications for rehabilitation. *Clinical Management in Physical Therapy*, *8*(1), 6-13.

Galantino, M.L. and Brewer, M., (1989, July 24). Peripheral neuropathies associated with AIDS: A case study in pain management. *Occupational Therapy Forum*, 11-13.

Galantino, M.L. and Spence, D., (1987, May). The role of physical therapy in the clinical management of AIDS patients. *Physical Therapy Forum (Western Edition)*, *6*(20), 1, 3-5.

Garcia, M.E., Collins, C.L. and Mansell, P.W.A., (1987). The acquired immune deficiency syndrome: Nutritional complications and assessment of body weight status. *Nutrition and Clinical Practice*, *2*(3), 108-111.

American Association of Immunologists (1989, March). Neuromuscular diseases of AIDS. Seventy-third Annual Meeting of the Federation of American Societies for Experimental Biology. New Orleans, Louisiana.

American College of Sports Medicine Guidelines for Graded Exercise Testing and Exercise Prescription (Second Edition). (1980). Author. Philadelphia Lea and Febiger.

Rigsby, L.W., Raven, P.B., Jackson, A.W., Dishman, R.K., and Berk, L.S., (1989, June). The effects of exercise and counseling on the physiological, psychological and immunological factors in HIV positive individuals. Presentation at the Department of Health, Physical Education and Recreation, University of North Texas, Denton, Texas.

Simpson, P., Bender, A., and Herman, S., (1986, June). Polymyositis in association with AIDS. Paper presented at the World Health Organization International Conference on AIDS. Paris, France.

Spence, D., Galantino, M.L., Mossberg, K. and Zimmerman, S., (in press). The effect of progressive resistance exercise on muscle performance and anthropometry in a select AIDS population. *Archives of Physical Medicine and Rehabilitation*.

Upledger, J.E. and Vredevoogd, J.D., (1983). *Craniosacral therapy*. Seattle: Eastland Press.

AIDS in a Correctional Setting

Victoria P. Schindler, OTR

SUMMARY. This article will provide current, relevant information on human immuno-deficiency virus (HIV) and Acquired Immune Deficiency Syndrome (AIDS) in the correctional setting. Issues pertinent to the correctional setting, such as HIV testing and confidentiality, transmission of the HIV virus in the correctional setting, and HIV related education will be explored. An occupational therapy program, outlining two separate programs for (1) those who are HIV positive and those who are diagnosed with AIDS and (2) those at risk for contracting the virus, will be described.

INTRODUCTION

Acquired Immune Deficiency Syndrome (AIDS) has presented several administrative and clinical management issues in our correctional facilities as well as financial, medical, and legal issues. There are a variety of reasons for this including the special needs of this group and society's views of this population.

The literature review addresses these issues and presents a current, comprehensive view of HIV infection and AIDS in the correctional system. This is followed by a description of an occupational therapy HIV/AIDS program in a forensic psychiatric facility. A review of the literature found no information on HIV/AIDS in a forensic setting. Therefore, since the forensic setting described is a maximum security setting which services inmates from the state, county and local jail/prison system, the pro-

---

Victoria P. Schindler is currently working as the Director of Rehabilitation Services at the Forensic Psychiatric Hospital, West Trenton, NJ. She is also the co-developer of the AIDS Program at the facility. Additionally, Ms. Schindler is a volunteer for the Hyacinth Foundation/New Jersey's AIDS Project, New Brunswick, NJ. In the past Ms. Schindler has worked with persons with AIDS (PWAs) in a variety of inpatient and outpatient settings and has presented at conferences and authored an article on the subject of AIDS.

gram described is representative of most HIV/AIDS programs in these settings.

THE CORRECTIONAL POPULATION

The current issues in the literature regarding this population address the following areas: (1) background regarding prisoners with AIDS (demographics, characteristics, and concerns unique to prisoners); (2) education; and (3) program development.

Incidence and Prevalence of HIV in Prisons

The first documented case of a prisoner with AIDS occurred in 1981 (Wormser, 1987). In a letter to the *New England Journal of Medicine*, Hanrahan, Wormser, Maguire, DeLorenzo and Gavis (1982) described cases of 7 inmates who, since 1981, developed opportunistic infections while in an upstate New York prison. Hanrahan's letter stated that the infections in the prisoners were probably part of the group of cellular immunodeficiency and unusual infections occurring in gay men and intravenous (IV) drug users and concluded that prisoners may represent a high risk group for the syndrome. Later, Wormser and his colleagues (Wormser et al., 1983) described in detail the cases of 7 previously healthy inmates in the New York correctional system who developed pneumocystis carinii pneumonia (PCP), all of whom denied homosexual behavior but did give a history of IV drug usage over a range of 7 to 25 years prior to incarceration.

Another study in the New York State Correctional System assisted in defining the early prevalence of the disease. All New York State prisoners who die during incarceration are required by law to undergo a postmortem examination. Review of these exams on 168 prisoners who died from nontraumatic cases during an approximate 5 year period preceding the first recognized case of AIDS in a New York State prison, failed to show a single case with findings which suggested AIDS. This retrospective study not only showed a historical perspective on the influx of AIDS in the New York state prison system, but it also helped establish AIDS as a genuinely new disease in this country. This was due to the assumption that if undiagnosed cases were occurring in the general population, they should also be occurring in the prison population due to the high risk behaviors among prisoners (Wormser, 1987).

The Middle Atlantic States (NY, NJ, PA) account for the majority of AIDS cases in correctional facilities. There is a particularly high incidence in the number of cases in inmates from the New York City and northern New Jersey area. The cases in this area and in the entire Middle Atlantic area are due to the increased use of intravenous drug use in this part of the country. However, as time progresses, AIDS cases in correctional facilities have increased in all regions and the distribution of cases is less uneven than it was several years ago. Additionally, incidence rates are higher in the correctional system than in the general population due to the concentration of persons with high risk behaviors (especially IV drug use) in correctional facilities (Hammett, 1988a).

HIV Testing and Confidentiality

The issues of HIV antibody screening and testing and confidentiality are highly controversial issues in the national justice system. Some of the issues involved in the debate include mandatory testing, accuracy of the HIV tests, the effect of testing on medical issues, and the extent of confidentiality regarding the results of the tests.

Currently, the Federal Bureau of Prisons has mandatory testing. Initially, the Federal system screened all new inmates but now only tests a random sample of 10% of incoming inmates and all inmates on release. An increasing number of state systems have instituted HIV antibody screening and testing programs, but the procedures and extent of testing vary widely, with some states linking results to individualized inmates. Because of the rapid turnover in city and county jail systems, there has been no institution of mandatory testing in these facilities (Hammett, 1988a).

The major controversy regarding testing is the effect of the results on inmate housing and the possibility of segregation of inmates according to their HIV status. This could be extremely detrimental if the HIV status resulted in two populations, with those testing positive isolated in one area of the prison, thereby promoting serious security problems and perhaps reduced inhibition to further transmit the virus. Those testing negative would be housed in the general prison population. Inaccurate test results or testing performed during the "window" phase, in which the person may be infected but may not yet show the antibodies to the virus, can lead to a dangerous situation.

All of this has led the Federal Bureau of Prisons to stop the policy of prisoner segregation although this policy does continue in some state correctional facilities. The new Federal policy calls for mainstreaming prisoners and segregating only those who are violent and assaultive and who create an actual risk of infection (Wormser, 1987, Hammett, 1988a, and Public hearing, 1989). Those in favor of segregation state that this method of housing protects prisoners with HIV/AIDS from physical injury or death inflicted by fellow prisoners (Wormser, 1987).

Other issues regarding HIV testing relate to the impact of this information on the medical aspects of HIV. Those against mandatory testing argue that it is unfair to subject inmates to mass testing and to stigmatize those who are HIV positive if there are no effective treatments or cures to offer them once a positive result is established. Those supporting mandatory testing argue that early identification of seropositive inmates promotes early, timely medical diagnosis and intervention, at least for opportunistic illnesses (Hammett, 1988a). The success of AZT in delaying the signs and symptoms of early and advanced AIDS related illnesses, as well as development of antiviral drugs with fewer side effects, may increase support for mandatory testing among inmate populations (Trenton Times, 1989).

The issue of confidentiality is linked to HIV testing centers and maintenance of confidentiality in a prison system. Those critical of mandatory testing believe that it is almost impossible to maintain confidentiality in a prison system. Proponents of mandatory testing argue that confidentiality can be maintained as long as care is taken to keep all information regarding HIV status in a secured area which is only for use by certain authorized personnel (Hammett, 1988a).

HIV Transmission in Correctional Facilities

The complex issue of HIV transmission in correctional facilities sparks much controversy since it alludes to security difficulties in the institutions.

Several studies have been conducted which point to low rates of transmission during incarceration (Kelley, Redfield, Ward, Burke, and Miller, 1986, NY State Commission of Correction, 1987, and Hanrahan et al., 1984). The belief is that the inmates brought AIDS with them, based on the idea that intervals between inmates entering the system and receiving a diagnosis of AIDS is generally much shorter than most estimates of the disease's incubation period (Hammett, 1988a). Ironically, it is also felt that incarceration may actually benefit some seronegative individuals by protecting them from HIV infection (Wormser, 1987).

The opposing view states that HIV infection can be transmitted through sexual activity and IV drug use which occurs in even the best managed correctional facilities. Proponents describe several factors of prison life which they believe support HIV transmission in correctional facilities. First, there have been known outbreaks of syphilis which suggest the occurrence of homosexual activity in prison (Wormser, 1987 and Hammett, 1988a).

Of particular interest is the extent to which homosexual activity among inmates is coerced. According to the Federal Bureau of Prisons, 9-20% of inmates are targets of aggressive acts during their imprisonment. However, less than 1% were actually found to be victimized (Hammett, 1988a). Other information supporting transmission in prisons points to the fact that many inmates have a history of IV drug use and that it is probably inevitable that at least some needle sharing takes place. Finally, tattooing and the sharing of razors are common in some correctional facilities and these activities can expose an inmate to the HIV virus (Hammett, 1988a).

Medical and Psychosocial Issues of HIV

A major issue in relation to medical and psychosocial issues of HIV is whether or not inmates receive the necessary care for this multifaceted syndrome. Investigators in the New Jersey Public Advocate Office of Inmate Advocacy state that many prisoners, especially those in the overcrowded county jails, are not being diagnosed or treated for AIDS related conditions for months after symptoms become obvious. This is contrary to state/federal law and to the missions of jails and prisons (Public Hearing, 1989). In fact, overcrowding of city jails has led to the discharge of inmates with HIV since there were no means for appropriate segregation and treatment (Manno, 1989).

Although there are still questions as to whether the most effective and efficient treatment is available and whether this should be conducted in a segregated or non-segregated atmosphere, medical and psychosocial services have been identified for this population.

The basic medical issues regarding HIV are similar both in and out of correctional facilities. Prompt detection and diagnosis of AIDS related conditions is needed for the most effective treatment. All correctional facilities conduct initial and regular physicals which support early diagnosis and treatment. The fact that these are done at regular intervals promotes earlier detection in the prison population than in the general population. Once an inmate is diagnosed with AIDS or ARC, regular follow up appointments are necessary since serious HIV related infections can develop rapidly. Many prisons which do not have the facilities or capacity to treat severely physically ill inmates often have a contract with a local hospital which has a medical ward for prisoners. In addition to prompt, effective treatment for the opportunistic infections, inmates should also be offered therapeutic medication to attack the virus itself (Hammett, 1988a).

Many of the psychosocial issues affecting civilians with HIV infection and AIDS also affect prisoners. Among these issues are HIV infection as a contagious disease and issues regarding homosexuality or drug abuse. These issues may be surfacing for the first time or may reappear as issues which have not been resolved. Persons with HIV infection and AIDS also must cope with declines in physical, psychosocial and cognitive functioning and may have their life roles severely or terminally interrupted (Schindler, 1988). Feelings of guilt, shame, fear, abandonment, anger and depression may surface at various stages of the illness (Hammett, 1988a and Schindler, 1988). Because of these feelings and the possible removal of support systems, psychological support and counselling is necessary for the prisoner with HIV.

Research in the Correctional Setting

Although the prison population does present its own needs medically and psychosocially, this population also provides an excellent resource for research with the goal of improved treatment and increased accuracy of statistical information. The prison population is a well defined group in which many factors can be controlled. For example, laboratory studies and medical examinations are always performed on admission and are conducted routinely during an inmate's incarceration. This provides opportunity for systematic retrospective review. Secondly, high risk behaviors, such as IV drug use and homosexual activity, are definitely decreased and hopefully interrupted during an inmate's incarceration. Restricted environmental exposure, which is an essential feature of prison life, allows for a more controlled, regulated environment. All of these factors make the prison setting an excellent site for research (Wormser, 1987).

EDUCATION AND TRAINING

Due to the potential for transmission of the HIV virus in the prison system and the positive effect of good health and medical habits on the impact of the HIV virus, education and training for both inmates and staff is the key tool to monitor the transmission and course of HIV infection.

Inmate Education and Training

Inmate education and training is usually viewed as a requirement in any prison setting. Ninety-six percent of the jurisdictions responding to the third annual survey offered by the National Institute of Justice (NIJ) in 1987 stated that they are currently offering or developing AIDS training/ educational material for their inmates (Hammett, 1988a). In 1986, the New Jersey Department of Corrections, in cooperation with the Department of Health, initiated an AIDS Education Program in the State Correctional System. This program was offered to all inmates who were due to be released on parole. It addressed issues such as safer sex, and risks of IV drug use, and offered information regarding HIV antibody testing and counselling sites. It was the first program of its kind nationally and reached over 2000 inmates in its first 7 months (Coye, 1987).

It has been more difficult to establish educational programs in the city and county jail systems due to the rapid turnover and increased crowding. Also, some county jails have reportedly treated the Surgeon General's report as contraband and have refused to deliver it to inmates (Public Hearing, 1989). In a 1985 National Institute of Justice survey, 73% of the city and county jail systems were providing AIDS education (Hammett, 1988a).

Most of the discussion regarding inmate education is centered around the content and method of teaching rather than the absence or presence of education. Training on HIV infection in seminar and discussion group formats provide the most effective means of training since they address the dissemination of current factual information and provide inmates with a timely and effective forum in which to ask and receive answers to questions. This may be supplemented with passive means of education, such as pamphlets and videotapes which, if used alone, may do more harm than good in that inmates may have questions and concerns without an arena to verbalize and discuss their needs (Hammett, 1988a). Educational content should address issues such as medical aspects of HIV, transmission of HIV, and prevention of transmission. The content should be factual and be conveyed in clear and simple terms understandable to the layperson.

Staff Issues and Education

Since a common behavior among inmates is assaultiveness toward fellow inmates and staff, the risks of contracting the virus through altercations with inmates who are HIV positive is a concern among staff members. Staff fear that behaviors such as biting, spitting, or throwing urine or feces may place them at risk. Managing inmates who have been involved in an altercation and are bleeding or restraining an inmate who is bleeding are two of the greatest fears of staff. However, 3 successive surveys conducted by the National Institute of Justice have failed to identify a single job related case of HIV infection or AIDS among correctional staff.

Staff need to be educated about the facts regarding transmission of the virus to allay unrealistic fears. For example, it is important to know that the HIV virus has been isolated in only very small concentrations in urine and saliva and not at all in feces. Most importantly, there have been no known cases associated with transmission of HIV through saliva or urine.

Additionally, for a staff member to be at risk for contracting the virus from an inmate who is bleeding, the inmate's blood would have to come in contact with the staff member's blood (Hammett, 1988b).

Several other issues, in addition to the fear of contagion, can influence a staff member's relationship with the inmate. Some of these issues include fear of dying, fear of overidentifying with the inmate, and homophobia (fear of homosexuality). Education regarding AIDS, peer support groups, and ongoing supervision can enhance a staff member's ability to recognize these issues and deal with them in an appropriate, productive manner. These forums can also enable staff members to ventilate fears and concerns associated with this challenging population (Schindler, 1988).

PROGRAM DEVELOPMENT

Program development for a correctional facility often focuses on two areas: (1) education, medical and psychosocial support services for those who are HIV positive and those who have developed ARC or AIDS and (2) education for those who are at risk for contracting the virus. The type of educational material presented will depend on the situation of the inmate. For those who are HIV positive and those with AIDS or ARC, education will focus on medical aspects of the illness with an emphasis on prolonging health, bolstering the immune system, and preventing transmission of the virus to others. For those who are at risk for contracting the virus, education will focus on prevention of transmission (Hammett, 1988a and Hein, 1989). Most correctional facilities require these two types of support services.

The program described below is one which has been instituted in a maximum security forensic psychiatric hospital.

Program Description

The Forensic Psychiatric Hospital is New Jersey's only maximum security forensic facility. It's responsibility is to provide a highly structured, secure and supervised environment for those who are impaired by mental illness, unable to control their behavior and have committed serious crimes. The therapeutic management process must be provided in concert with the legal justice system. Evaluation and intervention is provided in a setting in which the security aspect of the environment dominates.

The Forensic Psychiatric Hospital admits individuals from 21 county correctional facilities, 15 state correctional facilities and all city and municipal police authorities and state and county psychiatric hospitals. A total of 91% of the population is admitted from state and county correctional facilities. The population at the facility ranges in age from 18-65 with the majority of residents between the ages of 22-36 years.

Since the majority of residents are young men admitted from the state and county correctional facilities, the population is a cross-section of the correctional population at risk for developing AIDS. The two types of educational, medical, and psychosocial support services previously described have been instituted at the facility and incorporated into the occupational therapy program.

Occupational Therapy—
Individual Assessment and Intervention

The occupational therapist provides intervention to both of the populations described above (e.g., residents with HIV infection/ARC/AIDS and those at risk for contracting the virus). For residents with HIV infection and diagnoses of ARC or AIDS, the occupational therapist provides individual assessment and individual/group intervention.

The Model of Human Occupation is incorporated as a frame of reference for evaluation and intervention (Kielhofner, 1985). Assessment is comprehensive and includes an evaluation of the resident's motor, sensory/perceptual, cognitive, psychological and social skills. These areas are evaluated in regards to the resident's volitional system (personal causation, goals, and interests), habituation system (internalized roles and habits), and performance system (skills). The resident's current and expected environment and temporal adaptation are a focal part of the assessment. Physical needs which are unable to be addressed at the psychiatric facility (i.e., wheelchair prescriptions) are referred to the occupational therapy department in a local general hospital. The evaluation/intervention process will be illustrated in the following case study.

Case Study

L, a 40 year old divorced female with a long history of psychiatric illness and substance abuse, was admitted to a maximum security psychiatric facility from a county jail. L was admitted for an evaluation to determine her competency to stand trial on a charge of aggravated arson. Prior to incarceration in jail, L was living on the streets, supporting herself as a prostitute and regularly abusing IV heroin for 15 years.

On admission L presented with extremely bizarre, hostile and threatening behavior. She demonstrated increased psychomotor activity and was delusional about being pregnant. She was disheveled and emaciated and appeared much older than her stated age. Laboratory tests and evaluations were conducted, and L was diagnosed as HIV positive. Additionally, a CAT scan demonstrated a possible cerebral lymphoma. L stated she had lost 30 pounds in 2 months and continued to lose weight despite a diet supplemented by Ensure.

Occupational Therapy evaluation revealed L's goals, interests, roles, and habits were dysfunctional. Her most recent role was that of a prostitute and IV drug user, and she initially stated a goal to return to this lifestyle. Although she had marginal self care skills, they were not organized into habits. Further evaluation of performance skills revealed that L had a high school diploma but no work skills or productive work history. Her social behavior was loud, intrusive and sexually preoccupied. Her leisure interests focused on IV drug use, and she had no functionally appropriate leisure skills. Cognitively, she had an attention span of 5 minutes and subsequent lack of productive skills in decision making, problem solving and following directions. Psychologically, she denied her HIV status and was unable to utilize functional coping skills.

L was referred to a variety of individual and group occupational therapy programs. L began a cognitive retraining program to improve her basic work/task skills and to further evaluate dementia or organic disorders. L attended a social skills group to learn more appropriate methods to interact socially and to understand the life threatening impact of her sexually promiscuous behavior in social situations. The occupational therapist worked with L and the security staff to learn and incorporate daily self care habits in areas of diet, health, and hygiene. L needed to understand the importance of keeping herself healthy and drug free due to her now compromised immune system. L also attended a leisure interest group to explore and become comfortable with alternative methods to spend leisure time. All of these areas were significant in determining L's competency to stand trial and in preparing her to return to the jail.

Occupational Therapy — Educational Program

The occupational therapist participates in developing and co-leading an HIV/AIDS education program for the large group of residents who are at risk for contracting the HIV virus.

This educationally oriented program is provided in a group situation and is entitled "AIDS Education Group." The group is available to all residents who are able to attend to the task/discussion, can tolerate the presence of others, and show a need for basic education regarding the illness. The group meets for a 2 hour session once per week, and consists of 8-10 referred residents. The group is co-developed and implemented by the occupational therapist and the infection control nurse (Ferguson and Schindler, 1989).

The program consists of three major parts. A slide presentation of basic information on AIDS and a discussion with handouts address the following questions:

1. What is AIDS?
2. How does a person get AIDS?
3. How would you know you have AIDS?
4. What is the testing procedure for the HIV virus?
5. What is the treatment for AIDS?
6. How can I prevent myself and others from getting AIDS?

Following the discussion, patients watch a 40 minute video which portrays the lives of three individuals with AIDS who are in a correctional facility. The video follows the individuals through the course of their illnesses. The intention of this solemn, realistic view of the illness is to motivate the residents to take preventive measures in contracting HIV.

The residents then participate in a structured group activity designed to reinforce and evaluate their knowledge of the information presented. An example is an activity in which the residents are divided into two groups. Each group is responsible for developing 8-10 questions and answers to present to the other group. Then, each group alternates in asking the other group questions. The purpose of the activity is to assist the residents in recalling and integrating the material presented to them. Questions and discussion from the residents through the group session are encouraged (Ferguson and Schindler, 1989).

CONCLUSION

The purpose of this article was to present a view of AIDS in the correctional setting and to provide guidelines and an example for program development in this type of facility. Issues pertinent to this type of facility were explored. Some of the major issues facing the correctional setting today include prevalence of HIV, HIV testing and confidentiality, transmission of the HIV virus in the prison setting, medical and psychosocial issues regarding the illness, and staff and inmate education and training. Due to the highly structured and supervised nature of the correctional setting, it is an ideal environment to gather research on these topics which may ultimately benefit the entire public. An occupational therapy program description was provided which highlighted an evaluation and intervention

program for residents with HIV infection and those diagnosed with ARC
or AIDS and an educational program for those at risk for contracting the
HIV virus.

QUIZ

1. *List four of the most outstanding issues regarding AIDS in the correctional system.*
2. *List two reasons why AIDS may be more prevalent in the correctional system than in the general population.*
3. *Describe the major controversy regarding HIV testing in the correctional system.*
4. *What aspects of medical intervention in prisons can promote early detection and research into the AIDS illness?*
5. *What type of training is most effective for inmates?*

REFERENCES

New York State Commission of Correction (1987, Sept.). *AIDS: A Demographic Profile of NY State Inmate Mortalities, 1981-1986, Update*. Albany, NY: Author.

AZT can Prolong Lives of AIDS Patients. *Trenton Times*, Trenton, NJ, 8/16/89, A13.

Coye, M.J., (1987). *AIDS in New Jersey*. Trenton, NJ: Department of Health.

Ferguson, S. and Schindler, V., (1989). AIDS Education Group Protocol, Forensic Psychiatric Hospital.

Hammett, T., (1988a). *AIDS in Correctional Facilities: Issues and Options (3rd ed.)*. Washington, DC: National Institute of Justice.

Hammett, T., (1988b). AIDS and the Hospital Security Officer. *AIDS Patient Care*, 6/88, 38-40.

Hanrahan, J., Wormser, G.P., Maguire, G., DeLorenzo, L., and Gavis, G., (1982). Opportunistic Infections in Prisoners. *The New England Journal of Medicine*, 307: 498.

Hanrahan, J., Wormser, G.P., Reilly, A., Maguire, B., Gavis, G., and Morse, D., (1984). Prolonged Incubation Period of AIDS in IVDA: Epidemiological Evidence in Prison Inmates. *The Journal of Infectious Disease*. 150: 263-266.

Hein, K., (1989). The HIV Epidemic and Incarcerated Youth. *Correct Care*. Vol. 3, Issue 1.

Kelley, P., Redfield, R., Ward, D., Burke, D., and Miller, R., (1986). Prevalence and Incidence of HTLV-III Infection in a Prison. *Journal of the American Medical Association*, 256: 2197-2198.

Kielhofner, G. (Ed.), (1985). *A Model of Human Occupation – Theory and Application*. Baltimore, MD: Williams and Wilkins.

Manno, R., (1989, January 23). AIDS Poses New Dilemmas for County Jails. *Burlington County Courier Post*, Burlington County, NJ, 1A, A4.

New AIDS Drug set for Tests, (1989, June 6). *Trenton Times*, Trenton, NJ, A4.

Plan for Professional Services Manual, (1989, July). Forensic Psychiatric Hospital, PO Box 7717, West Trenton, NJ.

Policy and Procedure Manual, (1989, April). Forensic Psychiatric Hospital.

Schindler, V., (1988). Psychosocial Occupational Therapy Intervention with AIDS Patients. *The American Journal of Occupational Therapy, 42*: 507-512.

Taconic Correctional Facility, (1985). AIDS: A bad way to die (video). Bedford Hills, NY.

Transcription of Public Hearing before NJ State Assembly Health and Human Resources Committee to examine policy issues relating to AIDS. Trenton, NJ, 2/9/89.

Wormser, G.P., (1987). AIDS in Prisons. *AIDS and Other Manifestations of HIV Infection* (Wormser, G.P., Stahl, R., Bottone, E. eds.) Park Ridge, NJ: Noyes Publication.

Wormser, G.P., Krupp, L., Hanrahan, J., Gavis, G., Spira, T., and Rundles, S., (1983). Acquired Immunodeficiency Syndrome in Male Prisoners. *Annals of Internal Medicine, 98*: 297-303.

St. Francis Center:
One Organization Responds to AIDS

Margaret Edson

SUMMARY. The St. Francis Center in Washington, DC was founded in 1975 to provide support and guidance for individuals and organizations facing life-threatening illness and bereavement. The Center began seeing clients who were living with AIDS since 1983, and has expanded all of its services to include components specifically designed for people living with AIDS and organizations serving people with AIDS. This article describes the origins of the Center and reveals how the organization grew to meet the challenges of AIDS. The Center can be seen as an organizational model for other pre-existing institutions. Brief case studies demonstrate the activities and techniques of the Center's counseling, training and volunteer support programs as they help people with AIDS, their families and service organizations.

"Just rub my feet," a woman who was dying of cancer told the priest who had come to see her. He lay down his prayer book, and rubbed her feet while she talked. "I am dying, and I know it, and I want to be buried in a plain pine coffin." He assured her that he would honor this wish, and in doing so the St. Francis Center in Washington, D.C., was conceived.

TO FACE DEATH HONESTLY

"What this woman needed, what every one of us needs, is the opportunity to face death honestly," says Rev. William A. Wendt, the man who

Margaret Edson previously worked on the cancer and AIDS in-patient unit at the National Institutes of Health. She wrote and designed the St. Francis Center AIDS training manual, LIVING WITH AIDS: PERSPECTIVES FOR CAREGIVERS. The manual can be purchased for $9.95 (including postage) from the St. Francis Center, 5417 Sherier Place, NW, Washington, DC 20016.

founded the St. Francis Center in 1975 and still serves as Director. "She taught me the great lesson that has guided the Center since the beginning: We must be honest about death. People who are dying and bereaved teach us about death, and they teach us about life. We must listen to them, be loyal to them, and respect them."

When he visited other people who were dying or bereaved, he found that the best intentions of clergy, doctors, neighbors and family members were often misguided. Everyone was rushing to intervene and arrange, and the person at the center of activity was forced to be cheerful and grateful. Everyone had a grandiose, imposing plan for dealing with death, and the person who was dying wanted a simple ceremony under a tree.

Wendt soon had some pine coffins and ash-boxes made, and he began sitting quietly with people and listening to their stories, their fears and insights. If they mentioned death, he allowed them to continue instead of urging them on to safer subjects. If they said they were sad, he nodded and said, "Of course you are. He died and you miss him." In a death-denying society, he gave people a chance to be honest.

THE GROWTH OF THE CENTER

From meeting one dying woman's simple request, the St. Francis Center has grown since 1975 to become a source of guidance, information and support for people living with life-threatening illness and bereavement. And since early 1983, this community-based, non-sectarian, non-profit organization has changed and grown to respond to the needs of people who are living with AIDS and HIV infection, and their families, friends and caregivers. At present, the Center has a staff of four full-time and five part-time employees. Ten professional counselors work out of the Center, and see over 100 clients each month. Center training and education programs reach over 6000 people each year.

Originally, Wendt established the St. Francis Burial and Counseling Society. Its mission was to help people face death, by assisting with simple funeral and burial arrangements, and counseling people who were dying. It is important to remember that ideas which are widely circulated now—such as living wills, hospice care, dying at home, and personalized rituals—were only marginally accepted in the mid-1970s. To tell people that they had the right to disagree with the doctors, the clergy, and the funeral directors was considered subversive. To talk openly about death was considered, well, morbid.

Counseling: Free to Talk

In working with people at the time of death, it became clear that they needed help for a period of time before death and during bereavement. The counseling program was developed to include individual and group sessions with professional counselors for people in many different situations: those who had been recently diagnosed with a serious illness, their family members, people who were dying and their families, and people experiencing bereavement from a recent death or a death in the distant past.

The goal of the counseling program, from the beginning, has been to provide a safe forum for people to explore their feelings and to help them draw on their own strengths as they face such difficult times. While some mental health programs are designed to discover the sources of present conflicts through careful excavation of the remote past, grief and bereavement counseling enables the client to respond to a single, overwhelming circumstance.

The most troubling emotions to people who are ill and bereaved are often sadness, guilt, and anger. In counseling they are free to admit to these feelings, and to think through ways to deal with them. It is a great relief to people who are ill and bereaved to have their struggles acknowledged, their progress affirmed, and their setbacks understood. Professional counselors, free from the ties that constrain family and friends, are able to support the honesty that is so difficult for people who are ill and bereaved to find.

Training for Change

The St. Francis Burial and Counseling Society was formed to help people overcome an obstacle, the persistent denial of death and the denial of rights to people who were facing it. When the name was changed to the St. Francis Center, the mission was expanded to include teaching people to accept death as a part of life and to respect the rights and feelings of people who were seriously ill, dying, and bereaved.

The St. Francis Center's education and training program developed and taught a course for high school students called "Death and Dying: A Course About Life and Living." Training sessions were designed for health and social service professionals about issues of death and dying, including "The Needs of the Dying," "Family Issues," and "Grief and Bereavement." Community and religious groups received training in the theoretical and practical aspects of life and death issues. As the Center grew in experience and renown, the strategy shifted to training the trainers: instead of working with high school classes, the Center staff taught the teachers how to lead their classes in explorations of life and death.

The Volunteer Friends Program

To meet the personal and practical needs of people facing illness and death, a volunteer program was established in the early days of the Center's history. Volunteers were carefully trained to work individually with people and their families, offering support and assistance to help them through difficult times. People who might have felt uncomfortable with the formality of counseling preferred to talk openly with a volunteer from the community who was familiar with issues of illness and death.

From the beginning this program was designed to be flexible, with each volunteer responding to the specific needs of each client: some pairs of volunteers met for coffee with their clients, others telephoned frequently. The professional staff of the Center was always available as a resource for consultation with volunteers, and when a situation arose that was too difficult for a volunteer to handle, volunteers were able to make appropriate referrals.

THE BEGINNING OF AIDS

In early 1983, Judy Pollatsek, the Center's Associate Executive Director, attended a public forum sponsored by the Whitman-Walker Clinic, a small Gay and Lesbian health center in Washington, to discuss an unusual and devastating disease that was affecting Gay men. While expanding its own medical and social services to meet the threatening AIDS crisis, the Clinic began referring people with AIDS to Pollatsek and the Center for counseling. The St. Francis Center became the first counseling center in Washington to offer services for people with AIDS. As the Clinic developed a volunteer Buddy Program, Pollatsek began conducting a quarterly 20-hour training session focusing on issues of death and dying for new groups of buddies. As more and more health and mental health facilities, schools and community groups began to hear of AIDS, they requested information and training from the Center about the emotional aspects of life with AIDS.

During the years 1983-1986, the Center's stature grew as a resource for people living with illness and death. The staff and budget doubled. Some projects have been initiated that pertain only to AIDS, and some staff members have been hired to work exclusively in AIDS. At present, approximately 20% of the Center's clients and trainees are directly affected by AIDS. This percentage is expected to increase, but it is doubtful that it will exceed 50% of the total number of people served by the Center. The St. Francis Center is a community-based organization that existed before AIDS, will exist after AIDS, and devotes only a portion of its resources and efforts to AIDS. But, the Center has a deep commitment to bringing its unique services to people who are affected by AIDS.

COUNSELING PEOPLE WITH AIDS

The St. Francis Center's counseling program has always provided a safe place for people to explore the difficult emotions that come with illness and death. With AIDS, this is essential. To the overwhelming feelings that come with the diagnosis of any illness, AIDS brings with it a unique and complex set of emotions. People with AIDS are often shunned; they are most likely to have contracted HIV infection by doing something that is a private part of their lives; they are often young, and mourn the loss of their futures; they often have strained relations with their families; most people with HIV infection know several people who have died from AIDS; they know that chances are they, too, will die from AIDS.

In individual sessions, counselors allow people with AIDS to mourn for the cascade of losses they face, from the most simple pleasures to the deepest human needs. A counseling session is absolutely confidential, and a counselor meets each emotion not with judgment but acceptance. People with AIDS who are denied the chance to express and explore their feelings find that in counseling they are able to admit to emotions they had denied even to themselves.

Collaboration with other health care and human service providers is a critical component of our work. Therapists consult with medical teams, caseworkers, and occupational and physical therapists about a variety of issues and their impact on the clients' emotions, including: prognosis, values and goals, family patterns, financial resources, and care plans for the future. This is extremely important in a disease like AIDS in which the prospect of slow erosion of strength and independence must be faced by all clients. For example: a client reveals in counseling that eating in restaurants is an activity he used to enjoy and now misses because he has trouble managing the flatware. The client is referred to an occupational therapist for a consultation and is given special utensils. Thus this activity he grieved in counseling is restored by occupational therapy.

Tony

Tony was a powerful man. A high-ranking government official, he had a computer in his hospital room which linked him to his office network. He was a triathlete. With every dose of chemotherapy, he imagined that knights were on a crusade through his body, jousting with Kaposi's Sarcoma cells in mortal combat.

His counselor from the St. Francis Center met frequently with him in the last months of his life. He was from a large family, and his boisterous nature made him the one always cheering everyone else up. But his struggle with AIDS, combined with his perceived duty to be positive and enthusiastic, exhausted him. He found that he could let his guard down in counseling and that he could talk freely and honestly about how sad — and how scared — he was. With the freedom to face his emotions in counseling, he found a strength to be a speaker and advocate for people with AIDS until his death.

Partners

The partners of people with AIDS have their own set of needs. They face the challenge of caring for someone who may be seriously ill for months on end; they face the likelihood of bereavement; they feel they must be cheerful and helpful at all times; and they worry that if they get sick there will be no one to care for them. In counseling they are able to talk about these feelings, free from the fear of hurting anyone.

Families

Families of people with AIDS have their own complex emotions. A counselor who is familiar with AIDS and the issues that come with it is able to understand these emotions. It is interesting to note that family members feel especially comfortable seeking the services of the St. Francis Center, an organization that does not have an identity exclusively associated with the populations at risk for AIDS.

In addition to individual counseling for family members of people with AIDS, the Center conducts a free, bi-weekly, drop-in support group for people affected by AIDS in the family. The group provides a safe, understanding environment for family members, who are greatly appreciative of the chance to talk to other people in the same situation. The group is facilitated by two members of the Center staff on a volunteer basis. Confidentiality and anonymity are of supreme importance.

TEACHING ABOUT AIDS

The AIDS training program grew out of the challenges and successes of the Center's existing training program. The program works to increase the awareness, sensitivity and emotional stamina of individuals and organizations responding to the AIDS crisis.

Some of the training is designed to help schools, businesses and community groups understand the personal issues that lie behind the headlines about AIDS. The AIDS training coordinator meets in advance with individuals requesting the presentation, and they discuss the interests and needs of the group so that training is designed to respond to their needs. Frequently requested topics include "The Spectrum of HIV Infection," and "The Emotions of AIDS." An important component of these sessions has been the participation of a person who is living with AIDS, who speaks to the group and answers questions. A talk by a young person with AIDS makes a deep impression on school groups.

A critical part of all the Center's training about AIDS is the open admission of the fact that while AIDS is becoming a chronic illness, many people die because of it. The Center is proud to be associated with determined and courageous people with AIDS who continue to outlive their prognoses, but the fact is that some people with AIDS die, and everybody with AIDS knows it. The Center has always believed the honest discussion of death is far more beneficial than the supposed comfort of denial, and therefore, the Center's AIDS training program includes significant discussion of issues of death and dying.

Colleagues Helping Colleagues

A national trade union was becoming increasingly aware of the impact of AIDS on its members. The professional membership of the union had a large percentage of people at risk for contracting AIDS, and the administrators were anxious to learn about AIDS and how they could help their employees. Training about the transmission of HIV, emotional aspects of life with AIDS, and the impact of the death of a colleague on friends and co-workers, was designed.

The Center's trainer met with the group for two sessions, and discussed with them how to talk to colleagues who are ill, and what to say to the rest of the staff when one member becomes very sick and dies. The trainer listened to their sadness and frustration and reassured them that they are reasonable responses to a devastating disease that is touching so many of their friends. By encouraging them to be honest about AIDS, and honest about illness and death, the trainer showed them how to be supportive of their colleagues who are affected by the AIDS virus.

Weary Caregivers

Other training presentations focus on the needs of health care and social service professionals and volunteers working in AIDS. They face enormous stress, caused partly by the scope, complexity, severity and mystery of the disease, and partly by the emotions they have invested in the lives of their clients. Caregivers are taught to be detached, but they do become attached to the people they care for, and they are undeniably sad when a client becomes sicker or dies. The tension between what they are told to feel and what they actually experience may become a source of stress.

The Center's AIDS training program helps caregivers explore their emotions in their work in AIDS. They are allowed to reveal their feelings about working in a setting in which they watch so many young people die and are so unable to provide a cure, let alone a consistently effective treatment. There is frequently a great sense of relief when caregivers are finally able to admit and accept how they feel.

FRIENDS AND AIDS

The Center's volunteer Friends Program has been particularly attentive to the needs of people with AIDS and their family members. An important part of this program is the effort made to make things easier for families who have come from out of town to be with loved ones who have AIDS. This situation frequently accompanies a family crisis, such as a sudden hospitalization or very serious condition. Parents and siblings arrive at the airport and have nowhere to turn. Volunteers in the Friends Program often provide housing to these families on a short-term basis. They meet families at the airport, show them how to use public transportation, and have a cup of coffee with them in the hospital cafeteria.

The volunteers in the Friends Program fill the role of thoughtful neighbors in a strange city, but it is their training in issues associated with death and dying that is the most helpful to the families they serve. With these volunteers, family members can talk over the fears and feelings that are foremost in their minds. The volunteer is also aware of the needs of the person with AIDS and can help bring families together in these potentially divisive times. While several organizations provide companionship, only the Friends Program provides carefully-trained volunteers, at no charge, with whom clients can really talk about their losses and emotions.

Room for the Mother

A hospital social worker called to ask for a Friends Program volunteer for the mother of a patient with AIDS. The son was not expected to live more than a few weeks, and the mother refused to leave his bedside, sleeping in his room every night. The volunteer met with her in the hospital, and she agreed to go out for some lunch with him. In talking with the volunteer, she gradually realized that she could be away from her son and that it would even give her son a rest if she were not there. After a few days, the volunteer encouraged her to go home for the weekend, and when she returned, she stayed in her son's apartment and met frequently with the volunteer. When her son died, the volunteer helped her arrange for the funeral.

PERSPECTIVES FOR CAREGIVERS

The St. Francis Center staff has learned a great deal from clients in counseling and their caregivers in training. These lessons are included in the AIDS training manual published in the fall of 1989, entitled *Living with AIDS: Perspectives for Caregivers.* It is designed to help health care and social service professionals, community volunteers, family members and friends explore the emotional issues faced by people living with AIDS and HIV infection.

The book comprises six chapters: The Spectrum of HIV Infection, People Living with AIDS, Family Constellations, Weary Caregivers, Living and Dying, and Care and Loss. An annotated bibliography, and local and national resource guides are also included. Mathilde Krim, Founding Co-Chair of the American Foundation for AIDS Research, said of the manual, "This is a magnificent piece of work: concise, clear, practical, and yet so humane and sensitive."

LIFE, DEATH, AND HONESTY

AIDS has brought new challenges to the St. Francis Center, as it has to all service organizations in big cities. The Center was founded on a simple premise: death is a part of life, and people need to talk about it honestly. People who are dying have rights, and people who care for them have emotions. The Center is guided by the same philosophy in all aspects of its work with AIDS: death is a part of the experience of people with AIDS and those who love them. The Center offers these people a chance to talk about their feelings, and teaches their caregivers to do the same. It is the

Center's hope that in helping people face their most difficult emotions surrounding illness and death, they are free to participate more fully in their lives and their living.

QUESTIONS

1. Discuss this statement:
   People must be guarded from the harsh truth about death.
2. Discuss this statement:
   Thinking about death helps us think about life.
3. *What are some ideas and practices related to dying that have only recently become commonly accepted?*
4. *How do the emotional needs of partners of people with AIDS differ from the needs of the family members of people with AIDS?*
5. *What are some ways in which a trainer might be helpful to a group of co-workers of a person with AIDS?*
6. *Why do you think a trained volunteer might be able to make suggestions and have conversations with clients that a professional or a family member could not?*
7. *In what ways has the St. Francis Center changed to meet the AIDS crisis?*

Adult Day Care for People with Human Immunodeficiency Virus

Johnny Bonck, MS, OTR
Anne MacRae, MS, OTR

SUMMARY. The human immunodeficiency virus (HIV) adult day care (ADC) center is an important component in the continuum of care for the HIV ill client, providing therapeutic advantages to the client and administrative advantages to the community as it copes with the growing HIV epidemic. The HIV ADC center was designed using several models of adult day programs for developmental, psychosocial, geriatric and neuropsychiatric treatment. The HIV ADC client is typically in a non-acute phase of a chronic disability resulting from some combination of primary HIV pathology and secondary illnesses associated with the Acquired Immune Deficiency Syndrome (AIDS) and is in need of some level of rehabilitation. The HIV ADC client is typically a gay or bisexual male, a man or woman who is or has been addicted to intravenously injected drugs, or the sexual partner of someone in these groups. Programming addresses the psychosocial needs and daily realities of these populations. This article describes occupational therapy intervention focused on maintaining, restoring, or adapting functional skills, with special attention to the daily activities most affected by cognitive/perceptual dysfunction.

BACKGROUND ON DAY CARE

The social and health care system in the United States began to realize the need for long term and non-acute services for people with human immunodeficiency virus (HIV) illness not long after the beginning of the

---

Johnny Bonck is affiliated with the Occupational and Activity Therapy Department, Alta Bates/Herrick Hospital, Berkeley, CA.

Anne MacRae is Assistant Professor, Department of Occupational Therapy, San Jose State University, San Jose, CA.

195

epidemic (San Francisco Department of Public Health, 1989). This realization occurred as rehabilitation professionals were developing treatment protocols for acute care, extended care, and hospice care for people with HIV illness (Denton, 1987). Home care has become a standard component of the health care continuum (Bennett, 1988). Day programming is an area which complements home care and facilitates maintenance of the person living with HIV illness in the community.

For the purposes of this article, adult day care (ADC) refers to any program which provides services in a community based location to adults who are in need of supervision, assistance, or rehabilitation in order to maintain or improve quality of life. These programs also provide respite for the home caregiver, prevent or delay further inpatient treatment, and provide rehabilitative therapies, services, and counseling.

There are many reasons to develop day programs for the person living with HIV illness. First, there are clinical issues, especially the potent psychological benefits to most people of being at home rather than in an institutional environment (Rose & Catanzaro, 1989). Economic considerations are essential, since some communities are experiencing such a growth in the numbers of both geriatric and HIV clients that inpatient extended care capabilities are strained (Beresford, 1989). Outreach is essential, as in cases where the HIV-ill population is primarily comprised of IV drug users and their families. A community based program may be the only source of information and social and medical support available outside of an emergency room (Beresford, 1989).

There are two basic models for ADC services. One is the geriatric day health type facility which has been a part of the health care system for the growing geriatric population since the 1970s. The other is the community based day program for the psychiatric and developmentally disabled populations which presents an alternative to long term institutionalization. Within the geriatric model there are a range of programs and terminology varies. In Great Britain, there are geriatric day hospitals; in the United States a variety of terms are used including adult day health, medical day care, and residential health care facility nonoccupant services (Pomeranz & Rosenberg, 1985). Programs can be classified according to the level of care provided, the focus of the intervention, and the predominance of diagnoses and problems of the clients served. In general, programs are designated as social, maintenance or restorative in focus, either exclusively, or more commonly, in some combination.

The socially focused ADC program, the psychiatric day treatment program, and the day program for the developmentally delayed are similar in that the focus is usually on psychosocial rather than physiological intervention, but the diagnoses of the clients will determine the specific programming. Like the medical/geriatric model, these offer a daily meal and some form of therapeutic intervention through formal and informal programming. Transportation is a standard component of the medical/geriatric program and is sometimes available in the psychosocial model program. Because of the prevalence of neurological dysfunction in HIV illness, the day program for the treatment of dementia and other neuropsychiatric conditions is an excellent model for the HIV day program. The focus for this type of program is structure and continuity for the patient experiencing mental status changes.

The last decade has seen the development of Alzheimer's disease programs for maintenance of function and respite for caregivers (Cherry & Rafkin, 1988). Whether it is incorporated into a generic geriatric ADC program or is specialized and separate, the Alzheimer's ADC model that combines elements and approaches from the medical, geriatric, and neuropsychiatric models has much to offer the HIV ADC program for the client who is experiencing mental status changes due to dementia but who is otherwise relatively intact.

While they do not fit the strict definition of ADC used here, there are a number of community based and community organized drop-in centers that offer rest and relaxation for the person with HIV illness who is in need of a quiet, safe, and understanding place. Some of these centers offer meals, self healing groups, massage, and informal peer counseling as well as professional therapeutic and social services. They are often staffed largely by volunteers, many of whom are dealing personally with HIV illness. The successful ADC will incorporate the qualities of accessibility, flexibility, and community involvement that characterize this type of program. Because it is less expensive and requires less bureaucratic regulation, the drop in center is a possible starting point in the development of a comprehensive ADC program. Because of the potentially debilitating effects of HIV illness, the frequency of neurological involvement including dementia, the psychosocial and behavioral issues around role changes and addiction to substances, and the potential for return to higher function with rehabilitation, some combination of the above models will be ideal for the HIV day care program (see Figure I).

PROBLEMS ADDRESSED BY THE ADC
FOR HIV ILLNESS

Insofar as a person defines himself or herself by what he or she does, an enforced change in role can be devastating (Pizzi, 1988). Change and loss

FIGURE I

The Comprehensive Adult Day Care Model for HIV

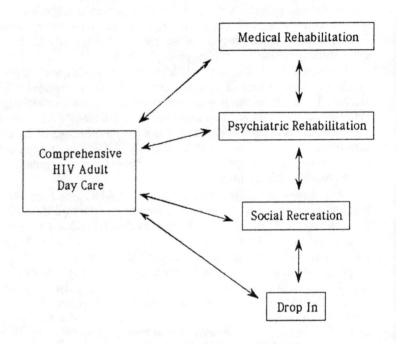

are constant and significant issues in the effort to live with HIV illness. Statistics indicate that a majority of people with HIV illness are in their most productive years (Pizzi, 1989). Changes in sexual behaviors, the need to replace dependent and addictive behaviors, changes in body image, the loss of the skills needed to survive on the streets, and the loss of spouses, children, lovers, and friends are major issues that will affect many. Regardless of vocational status, the person with HIV illness must confront the possibility or reality of radical decrease in energy level, the possibility of depending on others for assistance, the curtailment of activity and productivity, and the frustration and confusion of the unpredictable fluctuations in functional status (Pizzi, 1989). The day care center can provide a focus for adapting to new roles, can facilitate and teach coping skills, and can provide rehabilitation as appropriate.

PATHOLOGY

There is a large and somewhat daunting range of possible systemic non-neurological secondary illnesses that result from HIV illness but some of the main symptoms that affect function are fluctuating energy level, fatigue, weight loss due to gastrointestinal problems, and mobility problems due to joint pain and loss of muscle mass (Denton, 1987; Galantino & Levy, 1988).

HIV encephalopathy refers to the direct infection of central nervous system (CNS) tissue by the HIV (Levy & Bredesen, 1988). It is responsible for Acquired Immune Deficiency Syndrome (AIDS) dementia which can be a significant issue in a day program (see Table I). Opportunistic neoplasms and infections of the CNS can also result in mental status changes. Hemiparesis, hemiplegia, dysphagia, incontinence, peripheral neuropathies, and sensory loss (especially visual and tactile) are among the many symptoms of lesions or malfunction of nerve tissue that can be part of the HIV clinical picture (Bonck, 1987). There can be a significant overlap of maladaptive behaviors that pre-dated the HIV illness, behaviors due to the emotional stress of the illness, and behaviors that are frankly due to the neurotrophic activity of HIV, and these should be addressed in the treatment protocol. However, it is quite possible that a significant portion of social skills will remain intact in the client experiencing dementia and that these strengths should be used in implementing treatment.

TABLE I

Symptoms of HIV Dementia

Cognitive	Behavioral
slowing of mentation	apathy
short term memory loss	withdrawal
projective memory loss	disinhibition
decreased concentration	agitation
distractability	organic psychosis
confusion	manic states

CLIENT PROFILE

While there is no "typical" client, it is safe to characterize one who is most in need of a day program as relatively intact, mobile, not acutely ill, and in need of significant, if not constant, supervision due to mental status changes, such as forgetfulness, poor judgement, and problems with initiating and sequencing activities. One with major systemic illnesses in remission or under control but for whom residual neurological problems are an impediment to independent function is also characteristic of an ADC client. This client either needs a focus for social interaction due to an inadequate social network, or requires supervision during the day when the family/support system is at work or in need of respite from caregiver duties.

DEMOGRAPHICS

The demographics of the disease in North America are changing. For the first years of the epidemic, the disease mainly struck gay and bisexual males. Soon the majority of cases will be found among IV drug users (Heyward & Curran, 1988). The disease is increasingly found in heterosexual sex partners of IV drug users and the children of infected women. Unfortunately the disease is spreading disproportionately to the population size in the hispanic and black minorities (Heyward & Curran, 1988). Since the major coastal cities are the areas most heavily affected by the epidemic, chances are the ADC will be dealing with urban residents who come from some combination of these diverse sociocultural backgrounds. This diversity increases the challenge of creating meaningful programming.

People from disenfranchised populations tend to be suspicious of authority figures, including health care workers who are perceived to be part of "the system" (De La Cancela, 1989; Texidor del Portillo, 1988). This natural distrust can be overcome in a specific program by staffing personnel who either come from the minority population being served, or who at least have some understanding of and respect for the cultural issues of the client. Chemical dependency counselors are often clean and sober former users, and, as we mentioned earlier, the volunteer or professional staff may be dealing with their own HIV illnesses.

The heterogeneous client group might well be affected by communication issues, if not outright cultural clashes or prejudice. There has been debate about the integration of clients with HIV illness into health care programs versus establishing separate, specialized programs (Freeman,

1988). How the needs of specific sub-groups of clients with HIV illness will be served within the general HIV ADC program remains to be demonstrated. Programming decisions will be made according to available resources. At the very least, incidences of inappropriate behavior, racism, or homophobia need to be addressed on an ad hoc basis.

SUBSTANCE ABUSE

Based on the assumption that substance abuse interferes with the rehabilitation process, this issue must be addressed on an ongoing basis in programming for the HIV ADC program. Addiction presents a major barrier to the development of effective coping mechanisms. The drug addicted client may, in fact, be accustomed to the sick role due to a history of health problems and poor access to health care. Addiction is very difficult to control. The biological and psychological drive to satisfy the addiction can overwhelm any efforts to organize life around anything else (Zimberg, Wallace, & Blume, 1985).

Continued substance abuse is particularly an issue in a setting which focuses on psychosocial needs, especially if a client is not suffering from severe dementia and is independently mobile. If the program functions as a focus for social interaction, and the substance user is accustomed to a social life centered on using, then the temptation to get together and drug use will be substantial. One approach to the problem is to establish with the client a formal contract that is part of the initial orientation to the program specifying that substance abuse will not be tolerated, that a client with an identified problem must be actively engaged in some form of treatment for substance abuse, and that evidence of abuse will result in suspension from the program for some specified length of time. This kind of agreement does not guarantee the elimination of substance abuse as an issue in ADC. Ideally, there will be an outreach component built into an HIV ADC program through which clients who stop attending could be contacted, if not in person, then by telephone, by mail, or through other service agencies with which the client has contact (most especially that which is the source of income.) The availability of effective treatment programs will affect the success of the HIV ADC program.

EVALUATION

The occupational therapist can provide services in several capacities in the HIV ADC program according to licensing requirements and other administrative approaches. One possible role is that of case manager in which the therapist is involved in and responsible for the coordination of all aspects of the program for a number of individual clients. As a consultant, the therapist will design group and individual protocols for the various stages of the rehabilitation process, evaluate clients, and place them in the appropriate treatment track. The therapist can also provide direct patient care in group or individual treatments. In any capacity, formal evaluation, treatment planning, and implementation contribute to clear, measurable, and successful therapy. The protocol presented in Tables 2 and 3 is based on the occupational performance model and is influenced by developmental theory as well as the theory of human occupation (Hopkins & Smith, 1988). It is not within the scope of this article to provide detailed examples of all of the possible evaluation and intervention strategies outlined in Tables II and III. The discussion and examples are focused on issues that arise from HIV pathology in the community treatment setting.

Baseline Data

The baseline data will include some information about the clients premorbid functional level, main occupational roles, and family/support system specifics. It is important to learn as directly as possible from the client and the support system what roles (s)he has, what changes have occurred, and what coping mechanisms are used through direct observation and such assessment tools as the Moorhead Occupational History Interview (Moorhead, 1969).

The accustomed role of the heroin or cocaine user who is "in the streets" is to survive on a daily basis. The cycle of behavior of getting money for drugs, getting and using drugs, and getting food and a place to stay for the night is a totally consuming and very rigorous process, requiring considerable energy and skill. The debilitating effects of HIV illness can severely affect these behaviors and create a new kind of dependence (Hector Carillo, personal communication, September, 1989). On the other hand, a person who has been completely disenfranchised, homeless, and excluded from any effective social services, may find himself, because of an HIV diagnosis, suddenly with a regular "check" (source of income), a case worker, medical treatment, and a place to live; this will require some adjustment as well (Linda Gutterman, personal communication, September, 1989).

Interpersonal skills are significantly associated with the client's life roles and social skills. Mental status changes such as decreased frustration tolerance and attention span can sorely test social skills even as the client depends more heavily on them in the face of diminishing mental

TABLE II

Evaluation Procedures

Baseline Data (Premorbid Functional Level)

Psychosocial Issues

accustomed life roles

social support system

coping mechanisms

interpersonal skills

Stage in Disease Process

Medical status

acuity

medications

Cognitive/Perceptual Status

reality orientation

memory

organizational skills

visual perception

motor planning

safety awareness

judgement

Sensory/Motor Status

balance

gait

TABLE II (continued)

coordination

sensation/pain

muscle tone

strength

Activities of Daily Living (ADL)

grooming/hygiene

feeding

bathing

dressing

homemaking

community management

other self care regimes

(i.e. medications)

avocational interests

activity tolerance

"powers." Some clients, for example, may have difficulty tolerating group interaction regardless of premorbid interpersonal style.

The specifics of the support system of the HIV client are important to the effective assessment of safety in home and community management. Non-traditional family systems will be the norm in working with the HIV client. It is important to be as specific as possible rather than to make assumptions about the levels of commitment from roommates, lovers, and friends to provide ADL assistance for clients at home. In the absence of strong biological family ties, the client and his or her significant others may be without support for the emotional trauma of coping with a chronic disabling illness. On the other hand, a responsible network of friends may need to be included in all home and community management recommendations.

TABLE III

Treatment Procedures

Psychosocial Intervention

    expressive activities

    education of the support system

    stress reduction/relaxation techniques (massage, etc.)

    interpersonal skills development through group and individual social/task oriented

        activities

Cognitive/Perceptual Intervention

    neurodevelopmental techniques

    adapted activities

    compensatory techniques for maintaining memory, time management/organizational

        skills

TABLE III (continued)

Sensory/Motor Intervention

sensory stimulation

maintenance of strength, range of motion and endurance

tone normalization/neurodevelopmental techniques

functional mobility training (incorporating mobility and ambulation aids)

ADL Training

leisure time or avocational skills development

community management skills

home assessment

recommendations for adaptive equipment and assistive devices

self care re-training

attendant/caregiver training, education.

energy conservation

work simplification

206

The Disease Process

In general the ADC client will have developed some symptoms of secondary illness and/or will be exhibiting mental status changes. The ADC screening should provide a medical history. The acuity of the client is important. Significant fluctuations in functional status can affect participation in the program, and these need to be monitored for diagnostic purposes. Many of the treatments for HIV related illnesses produce side effects or involve invasive techniques (such as central line therapy) which will affect the client's functional status. Many drugs, especially neuroleptics, have a more potent effect in the client whose central nervous system (CNS) is already compromised by factors such as HIV illness. A client's taking of psychotropic medications may be, but is not always, an indication of a pre-morbid psychiatric history. Psychotropic medications have been shown to be effective in some cases of HIV related reactive psychiatric conditions (Perry & Jacobsen, 1986), and antidepressants seem to alleviate some of the pain and depression associated with peripheral neuropathies.

Cognitive/Perceptual Status

Due to the prevalence of HIV dementia, cognitive assessment is vital. Many clients will identify cognitive changes as a problem although an accurate self assessment of mental status changes is rare. Denial of these changes is not uncommon. Thus, therapist observation and interview of the support system will provide more accurate assessment. Dilley, Boccellari, and Davis (1989) have explored the pros and cons of the Mini-Mental Status Examination as a tool in HIV evaluation. Claudia Allen's Assessment of Cognitive Levels and Routine Task Inventory (Wilson, 1985) can be adapted to HIV illness. Ongoing objective assessment is important due to fluctuations in mental status associated with HIV. This is especially true for clients on life sustaining drugs such as AZT. AZT has demonstrated improvements in mental status in people with HIV dementia (Schmitt, Bigley, & McKinnis, 1988).

Sensory/Motor Status

Sensory/motor deficits can be disabling in HIV illness. Decreased strength and endurance, fine motor deficits, and decreased range of motion of the lower extremities due to peripheral neuropathy or edema are frequent problems that can produce functional deficits.

Activities of Daily Living (ADL)

As stated earlier, the mental status changes of HIV dementia will be significant in the areas of time management, task organization, initiation, sequencing, and safety at home and in the community. Medications to be taken at home are extremely important and become part of the client's routine. Direct observation of ADL will reveal information that the client cannot or does not wish to report on, and will have an impact upon the treatment plan for both the client and the therapist.

TREATMENT PROCEDURES

The rehabilitation process can be organized into three phases or approaches. The maintenance approach is appropriate for the client who is debilitated and for whom the prognosis is too poor to assume that the restoration of function is either practical or even possible. This client benefits from interventions designed to maintain remaining functions. The next category is the compensatory approach which is appropriate when the client is not able to regain function without adaptation of the environment or of methods by which tasks or behaviors are accomplished. The third approach is the restoration approach, whereby the client can and will regain function that has been affected by the disease process. In practice these three approaches are often used in combination. Temporary compensation techniques and adaptive equipment, for example, will be appropriate for the individual who is gaining strength and whose system is recovering from a secondary opportunistic condition, facilitated by a graded rehabilitation program. The client's psychosocial status might require an ongoing supportive group process to maintain emotional balance. These distinctions can greatly facilitate effective activity analysis and activity planning, and provide guidelines for grouping clients at their most appropriate functional levels.

Psychosocial Intervention

The ADC program provides ample opportunity for the client to re-establish healthy interpersonal skills needed to maintain healthy interpersonal relationships amid the stressors of HIV illness. Education in effective communication and stress reduction techniques and the opportunity to vent feelings in a positive and supportive environment are important treatment techniques.

Cognitive/Perceptual Intervention

A successful program of compensation and retraining for cognitive deficits such as one that allows the client to perform basic home and community management tasks safely and efficiently in spite of the memory loss and disorientation of HIV related dementia. It may well be the single most important contribution of an occupational therapy protocol to an ADC program.

Sensory/Motor Intervention

Established sensory/motor intervention strategies are modified according to the ongoing status of the HIV client. Paresthesias of the lower extremities and hypersensitivity to moderate or deep pressure are two symptoms of secondary illness that may affect functional balance training or the neurodevelopmental rehabilitation techniques of Brunstromm, Rood, and Bobath (Huss, 1988).

Activities of Daily Living Training

ADL training of the HIV client will be affected most significantly by neurological issues and success may well depend on the effectiveness of cognitive compensation/adaptation schemes. Medication regimens are often of particular importance because of the quantity of medications required to control chronic secondary conditions. Pre-set medication containers, timers, and enlarged and customized daily written schedules are examples of resources that can be adapted to the needs of the person with HIV illness. Effective and realistic education about safer sex techniques and the relationship between HIV infection and the sharing of hypodermic needles is an extremely important component of the HIV client's occupational therapy ADL training program.

CONCLUSION

Living with HIV illness rather than dying of AIDS is the wave of the future. To some, living with HIV illness means surviving difficult day to day experiences of fear, guilt, poverty and addiction. To some, it means embracing a proactive model of wellness, self-awareness, and growth. To all, it means coping with the reality of changing life roles and the possibility of facing limitations in accustomed daily activities. This article has suggested ways in which rehabilitation services and occupational therapy in particular can facilitate coping and minimize limitations as part of the community based Adult Day Care facility.

STUDY GUIDE QUESTIONS

1. *What justification is there for developing non-acute care services like Adult Day Care to treat a fatal, terminal illness like AIDS?*
2. *True or false: the ADC is appropriate for maintenance level clients only, and clients with significant rehabilitation potential should be referred to outpatient rehabilitation therapy.*
3. *If HIV illness affects the immune system, then why is dementia the focus of treatment?*
4. *Are health care workers in an ADC for HIV illness more likely to develop one of the rare secondary illnesses associated with AIDS?*
5. *True or false: the HIV client will often retain social skills even when suffering from HIV dementia.*
6. *True or false: although the disease was first identified in North America in gay and bisexual males, this population now comprises a tiny minority of cases.*
7. *Is it important that all HIV ADC clients be free of substance abuse?*
8. *True or False: It is recommended that because of the instability of the lifestyles of most people with HIV illness, the occupational therapy evaluation process should focus on direct observation and client interview for information.*
9. *What is the value of a detailed functional evaluation for a disease process that fluctuates so unpredictably?*
10. *True or False: The treatment of cognitive/perceptual dysfunction of the HIV client is successful only insofar as new learning is still possible.*

STUDY GUIDE ANSWERS

1. Answer: AIDS is just one phase of a chronic condition called HIV illness. Acute hospitalization in the treatment of HIV illness should be minimized for financial as well as therapeutic reasons.
2. Answer: False. Depending on licensing and program design, ADC can provide a full range of rehabilitation services to appropriate clients, and different levels of acuity can be accommodated in one center by grouping patients accordingly.
3. Answer: The two pathological processes in HIV illness are the dis-

ruption of the immune system due to the destructive action of the HIV, and the direct attack by the virus on tissue of the central nervous system. Dementia can be the result of either or both of these.

4. Answer: Only if they are HIV infected themselves or have otherwise seriously compromised immune systems. Refer to the terms *recrudescent* and *ubiquitous* in the text.

5. Answer: True, and this is an excellent means of facilitating maximum interpersonal skills and adaption to new roles.

6. Answer: False. Predictions are that eventually the IV drug using population will outnumber other at-risk groups in North America. There are still many gay and bisexual men with HIV illness who will be treated in ADC.

7. Answer: It is important to establish clear policies to deal with substance abuse, but relapses in sobriety and use should not permanently disqualify a client from participation.

8. Answer: False. Many clients will have strong and active, if nontraditional, support systems that will be involved in all aspects of care.

9. Answer: In addition to the need for evaluation in treatment planning, a functional baseline is important to monitor the effectiveness of treatment and to provide input to the diagnostic process which often depends, in the absence of laboratory tests, on careful observation of symptoms.

10. Answer: False. Adaptation and compensation for skills that are no longer intact is a major focus of occupational therapy intervention.

REFERENCES

Bennett, J., (1988). Helping people with AIDS live well at home. *Nursing Journal of North America*, *42*(8), 116-123.

Beresford, L., (1989, April 27). Adult day care for people with AIDS. *Long Term Care Management*, *18*(9), (Special report insert).

Bonck, J., (1987, September). The neurological sequelae of AIDS: Treatment issues for occupational therapy. *Physical Disabilities Special Interest Section Newsletter*, pp. 1, 6, 7.

Cherry, D.M., & Rafkin, M.J., (1988). Adapting day care to the needs of adults with dementia. *Gerontologist*, *28*(1), 116-120.

City and County of San Francisco Department of Public Health, (1989). *Report to David Werdegar, MD, MPH, Director of Public Health, from the Committee for Non-Acute Services for Persons with AIDS*.

De La Cancela, V., (1989). Minority AIDS prevention: Moving beyond cultural perspectives towards sociopolitical empowerment. *AIDS Education and Prevention, 1*(2), 141-153.

Denton, R., (1987). AIDS: Guidelines for occupational therapy intervention. *American Journal of Occupational Therapy, 41*, 427-432.

Dilley, J. W., Boccellari, A., & Davis, A., (1989). The use of the Mini-Mental Status Exam as a cognitive screen in patients with AIDS. Poster presentation, *Fifth International Conference on AIDS, Montreal, Canada*, abstract, p. 384.

Freeman, I., (1988). Caring for persons with AIDS in geriatric nursing homes. *Health and Social Work, 13*(2), 157-8.

Galantino, M., & Levy, J., (1988). Neurological implications for rehabilitation. *Clinical Management, 8*(1), 6-13.

Heyward, W., & Curran, J., (1988, October). The epidemiology of AIDS in the U.S. *Scientific American*, pp. 72-81.

Hopkins, H., & Smith, H., (Eds.). (1988). *Willard and Spackman's Occupational Therapy* (7th ed.). Philadelphia: Lippincott.

Huss, A. J., (1988). Sensory motor and neurodevelopmental frames of reference. In H. Hopkins, & H. Smith (Eds.), *Willard and Spackman's Occupational Therapy* (pp. 114-126). (7th ed.). Philadelphia: Lippincott.

Levy, R., & Bredesen, D., (1988). Central nervous system dysfunction in acquired immunodeficiency syndrome. *Journal of Acquired Immune Deficiency Syndromes, 1*(1), 41-64.

Moorhead, L., (1969). The Occupational History. *American Journal of Occupational Therapy. 23*, 331.

Perry, S., & Jacobsen, P., (1986). Neuropsychiatric manifestations of AIDS-spectrum disorders. *Hospital and Community Psychiatry, 37*(2), 135-142.

Pizzi, M., (1988). Challenge of treating AIDS patients includes helping them lead functional lives. *O.T. Week, 2*(32) pp. 6,7,31.

Pizzi, M., (1989, February). Occupational therapy: Creating possibilities for adults with HIV infection, ARC, and AIDS. *AIDS Patient Care*, pp. 18-23.

Pomeranz, W., & Rosenberg, S., (1985, Spring). Developing an adult day-care center. *The Journal of Long-Term Care Administration*, pp. 11-22.

Rose, M.A., & Catanzaro, A.M., (1989). AIDS caregiving crisis: A proactive approach. *Holistic Nursing Practice, 3*(2), 39-45.

Schmitt, F.A., Bigley, J.W., McKinnis, R., (1988). Neuropsychological outcome of Zidovudine (AZT) treatment of patients with AIDS and AIDS related complex. *New England Journal of Medicine, 319*, 1573-1578.

Texidor del Portillo, C., (1988). Poverty, self-concept and health: Experience of Latinas. *Women and Health, 3*(4), 229-242.

Wilson, D.S., (1985). *Cognitive disability and routine task behaviors in a community-based population with senile dementia*. Unpublished master's thesis. San Jose State University, San Jose, CA.

Zimberg, S., Wallace, J., & Blume, S.B., (Eds.), (1985). *Practical approaches to alcoholism psychotherapy* (2nd ed.). New York: Plenum Press.

Gay Grief:
Issues of Love, Loss, and Loneliness

Diane Okoneski, MSW

SUMMARY. This article is intended to provide an overview of the special needs for individuals who are gay and bereaved. Also included is a personal account from a lover whose partner died of AIDS. The intent of this article is to increase the level of understanding and sensitivity of practitioners who will be assisting persons affected by Human Immunodeficiency Virus (HIV).

INTRODUCTION

Acquired Immune Deficiency Syndrome (AIDS) has affected all segments of our society. However, the gay community has been particularly devastated by the number of deaths since the beginning of the epidemic.

Because society conditions its members to feel apprehensive toward those who lead alternative lifestyles, it is more difficult for gay men . . . to receive support while they mourn their loss. Society does not sanction intimate, same-sex relationships; yet it is the lack of sanction for this type of relationship that prolongs the grieving process. (Siegal & Hoefer, 1981, p. 518)

When The NAMES Project AIDS Memorial Quilt was displayed in

Diane Okoneski is a licensed clinical social worker presently at the Burgess Clinic, Children's National Medical Center, 111 Michigan Avenue, N.W., Washington, DC 20010. She has worked extensively with both adults and adolescents with AIDS. She has facilitated support groups for individuals, couples, and families relating to HIV/AIDS issues. She is also in private practice specializing in HIV-related counseling.

This is dedicated to a dear friend who contributed the "case study" portion of this article. It was his personal decision to share with us a most intimate part of his life so that others may learn to see the human element in AIDS.

Washington, D.C., during the fall of 1989, it contained almost 11,000 panels. It is a handmade memorial of overwhelming proportion that vividly symbolizes many themes. The individually sewn panels celebrate the life of each man, woman, and child who has died of AIDS. The collective panels, sewn together, present a grim reminder of the devastating effect this disease has had on our society. It is a very public display by thousands of strangers who have been united by the quilt to express both their love and sorrow. For some, however, it may be the only means of publicly acknowledging their grief. Many of the panels contain only a first name to acknowledge a loved one. A panel with

> The name 'Michael' is written on one side, but on the other side where his last name should appear, there is a gaping hole. His surname was cut out, literally by his parents, when Michael's lover showed them the memorial he had made for their son. (Ruskin, 1988, p. 78)

Regrettably, we are now a decade into this epidemic and the stigma of AIDS still exists. People with AIDS and those who care about them continue to be subjected to immeasurable isolation and rejection. Since the beginning of the AIDS crisis, the majority of cases diagnosed have been gay men in their twenties and thirties (Centers for Disease Control, 1989).

GAY GRIEF AND BEREAVEMENT: AN OVERVIEW

Gay communities across the country are witnessing ongoing devastation in their numbers.

> Not only are gay men losing those with whom they have shared strong emotional ties, but they are also losing acquaintances, role models, and co-workers at a very fast rate. The community life which they so recently created, or moved to the city to take part in, has undergone extreme and rapid changes as men have adapted to losses and brace themselves to experience more. (Dean, Hall & Martin, 1988, p. 55)

It is not uncommon for a gay man to know a few, a few dozen or a few hundred people who have died of AIDS. Thus gay men are mourning the deaths of their lovers, friends and community. These serial deaths and multiple bereavements are a common element in gay grief. Additionally, the threat of HIV infection that is widespread throughout the gay community creates additional stress. Dean et al., (1988) found "The subjective sense of threat associated with AIDS stems largely from the lack of clear answers about why one person becomes sick while another does not . . ." and ". . . problems generated by actual losses, anticipated losses, and hardships due to AIDS . . ." (p.54) increases ones sense of vulnerability and intensifies their feelings of grief.

The discrimination that gay men receive in our society has been widely documented.

> The lack of resources designed for gay people creates an even more difficult situation. When one is gay and lives in a community where homosexuality is not considered a human right, where does one seek solace? She or he cannot go to a priest because gays are considered sinners. Gays may not be able to go to a doctor, lawyer or work supervisor for fear of exposure, a potential jail sentence, loss of a job or status in the community. Nor can they expect to get support from their families for fear of rejection. (Siegel & Hoefer, 1981, p. 522)

A diagnosis of AIDS has often been the time that gay men have "come out of the closet" (identified themselves as being gay) to their families and friends. Their reactions, if not accepting or supportive, can create emotional pain and indignity for the gay couple and the bereaved lover. Unless a durable power of attorney has been prepared, the biological family has the final word on decisions, such as medical care for the person with AIDS. Regardless of how long a gay couple has been together these decisions can be made with or without including the lover.

If no will has been drawn up, the lover has no legal claim to any possessions shared by the deceased — sentimental or otherwise — if the family so chooses. Many persons with AIDS and their lovers have planned the funeral or memorial services and burial arrangements. However, there are many instances where families have forbidden lovers from attending the service, refused to disclose the nature of death to relatives, and never acknowledged that their son was gay. Even with prior planning, many times "Funeral arrangements and estates often were disputed. . . . This conflict made it more difficult for the significant others, some of whom were the primary caregivers, to cope" (Greif & Porembski, 1988, p. 261).

Gay men who are caring for someone with AIDS and who could be HIV positive themselves experience very high levels of emotional stress; they need to share their feelings with others.

> Not only is the significant other facing the probable terminal condition of a loved one, he or she also is facing what many persons perceive to be the stigma of AIDS coupled with homosexuality. . . . These issues are difficult for many to face and often result in the significant other being secretive about the diagnosis and condition of the person with AIDS. (Greif & Porembski, 1988, p. 259)

As one lover stated, "I felt so cheated not being able to tell anyone at work about "D," who he really was and how I cared for him. When he died I was devastated. My co-workers knew something was wrong but I was so afraid to tell them I was gay. So I said my brother had died, but it wasn't that at all."

Family and friends may provide little support to a person with AIDS and one's lover because of a fear of contagion and the perceived stigma associated with knowing someone with AIDS or who is gay. If a gay couple decides to limit the knowledge of the diagnosis to a few individuals, this element of secrecy creates its own cycle of isolation.

> When a spouse dies, the surviving spouse undergoes a transition to the role of 'widow' or 'widower.' That role, however vague, has a certain status that is recognized by the larger community. It carries legal and social rights. For example, bereaved spouses may be permitted time off from work, they are excused from certain social responsibilities, and they are permitted a wider range of emotional expression. (Doka, 1987, pp. 461-462)

The mental health professionals traditionally have been the source of support for gay men. As a result of the AIDS epidemic, there has been a surge in the number of support groups which address a variety of needs. These groups are usually geared toward specific populations, such as significant others, HIV positive persons, the worried well, couples, people with AIDS, and the bereaved. Groups offer a safe and nonjudgmental environment for members to talk about their experiences. Support groups provide members the benefit of both listening to others and sharing one's own experience. It also provides an opportunity to meet other people and expand one's social network. Additionally, the recently bereaved members of the group benefit from the experiences of other group members further along in the grieving process.

Bereaved lovers may also choose individual counseling to process their grief. Many people feel their pain is too private to be discussed in a group and are not emotionally ready to hear other persons' accounts and provide support to them. Their physical and emotional energies are so strained that they need personalized attention. However, whether someone chooses to join a group or to receive individual counseling, the issues addressed will be similar. It is crucial for individuals to have an opportunity to talk through their pain about their loss. "Homosexuals grieve over their partner's death as much as heterosexual people, but public prejudice often forces them to hide the nature of their relationship and suffer in silence" (Jones, 1988, p. 55).

While there are many descriptions of grief and bereavement available, the following one is particularly expressive in describing the pain and loss people experience.

> The death of a loved one is the most profound of all sorrows. The grief that comes with such a loss is intense and multifaceted, affecting our emotions, our bodies, and our lives. Grief is preoccupying and depleting. Emotionally, grief is a mixture of raw feelings such as sorrow, anguish, anger, regret, longing, fear, and deprivation. Grief may be experienced physically as exhaustion, emptiness, tension, sleeplessness, or loss of appetite. Grief invades our daily lives in many sudden gaps and changes, like that empty place at the dinner table, or the sudden loss of affection and companionship, as well as in many new apprehensions, adjustments, and uncertainties. . . . Hence to grieve is also 'to celebrate the depth of the union. Tears are then the jewels of remembrance, sad but glistening with the beauty of the past. So grief in its bitterness marks the end . . . but it also is praise to the one who is gone.' (Tatelbaum, 1980, p. 7)

Mental health, health care and other professionals can best serve persons with AIDS, and their lovers, families and friends by being sensitive, compassionate and understanding. It would be helpful for them to be aware of their own biases, prejudices and unresolved issues about sexuality, homosexuality, religion and death. The client relationship needs to be a trusting one. If the above elements are not present it could jeopardize any sort of healthy outcome. Therefore, practitioners will be most successful when they are honest with themselves before beginning interventions with clients whose situations they may be uncomfortable with.

> Clinicians need to be aware of and accept homosexuals . . . lifestyles as well as knowledgeable about grieving procedures before engaging in a therapeutic relationship with gay bereaved individuals. . . . there is still little awareness of the specific problems homosexuals encounter and society has few structures to deal with them. Homo-

sexual . . . couples who mourn their mates need to be seen and see themselves as worthy of support. (Siegel & Hoefer, 1981, p. 524)

ISSUES ADDRESSED IN GAY BEREAVEMENT COUNSELING

There are a range of topics to discuss with a bereaved lover. This section will highlight the themes that frequently are addressed when counseling the gay bereaved.

For some individuals it is helpful to begin with the events that led to the diagnosis of HIV or AIDS. This discussion will provide details of prior HIV status. For example, was either partner ever HIV tested, and if so, how did this decision and its implications affect their relationship? Who was told of the diagnosis, and what were the reactions? The decision of who or who not to tell about the diagnosis is not always mutual, and secrecy can create many difficulties. What affect did the diagnosis have on friends and family? Specifically, who was supportive and who was not? How was the situation handled with employers and co-workers? Was the gay relationship validated? For some lovers it will be important to receive acceptance of the relationship from the counseling session if they did not have it before.

Often times lovers need to discuss changes that occurred in their relationship after the diagnosis and to discuss how the pressures from the illness affected communication between the couple. Did the relationship become closer or move further apart; was suicide ever discussed; and what changes occurred involving habits, routines and roles? Has the lover discussed any legal, financial or insurance problems that developed? Has a will, living will or durable power of attorney been discussed or prepared?

Some people will need to talk about their lovers' deaths, including a discussion of whether or not they were present at the time of death and if not, how they were notified; what arrangements were made for a funeral, memorial service, burial or cremation; and the dynamics with the couple's friends and family, that is, how the lover was treated. It is also important for bereaved lovers to express any regrets with which they may be struggling. Lovers also need to share memories that reflect upon happier times during their relationship.

When a partner dies it is very difficult to begin to rebuild one's own life. The gay bereaved have specified the following topics as being of particular concern: their HIV status, their lovers' estates; possibly relocating; making a quilt panel; dating; sexuality; holidays; vacations and their new identity as single, bereaved gay men.

CASE STUDY:
A BEREAVED LOVER'S STORY

A partner who lost his lover to AIDS describes his experience in dealing with this disease.

"It has been ten months since R died. They say the first year is the hardest, and I believe it is. I can't wait for it to be over, just to have it behind me. I talk to R everyday and this helps me get through. I'm just beginning to have a sense of my own life. You can't pressure yourself, it has to come naturally. There's no way to get rid of the sad, lonely feelings. They don't ever go away, but you learn to deal with them in a healthier way as time goes on. This experience was a part of my life that changed my life. The experience R and I shared has made my life much richer, and as a result I understand the phrase 'to love is to let go.'

"When this disease impacts on a couple, one of two things will happen. Your relationship will either grow apart or become closer; it does not stay the same. When R was diagnosed with AIDS, our relationship was at a point where I could have walked away. But I did not. He was someone who cared a great deal about me, and I felt there was a need for me to be there. Faith is what our whole relationship was about. Faith is in not knowing. When you really care about someone it does not matter what will happen. What matters is your time together and the quality of that time. I would rather have a meaningful relationship with someone for three days than a meaningless relationship of 100 years. The amount of time is not what you celebrate.

"When R died on December 3, 1988, he had gone full circle in his life. We had learned about love and had experienced so much growth in his last years. In some ways I can see why God took him—he didn't have much else to live for. He had gotten all the good stuff, the really important things in life. Sure, if he had lived there were many good things he could have done. But R was fortunate to see the true value of life, love, respect and caring. He knew what it meant to take love, what it meant to give, and what it meant to be unselfish and to let go. He had carried around a lot of emotional baggage in his life but he also did a lot of work in his last few years. He died very peacefully, and I know in my heart and in reality he led a full life.

"R and I met July 4th weekend in 1986. It was a relationship that was right from the start. He was bright, attractive, and had a good sense of humor. But there was an innocence, a lack of sophistication about his demeanor that made him appear flip, separate and aloof. I sensed he was not comfortable with most people, very insecure, but this was endearing to me, a real mix of qualities. At that time, I was beginning to take better care of myself and my emotions. I had developed a better sense of self. It was a perfect time for both of us.

"R was a doctor at a local hospital and had treated some patients with AIDS. He also did volunteer work at the local AIDS service agency. I had my own business and also had done volunteer work as a buddy at the same agency. I am gay and very proud of who I am. I have a very loving and supportive family, and they were of great comfort to me throughout this experience. R was not 'out' at work and as a result had two circles of professional friends. One circle knew he was gay, and the other did not. His sister, L, who lived out of town knew. They loved each other very much and she was a tremendous support to us both. She continues to be a great support to me to this day.

"As our relationship developed, we decided to move in together in March of 1987. At that time, I had become somewhat suspicious of his health status. He had been tested before we met and knew he was HIV positive. I did not know my status at that time. However, when I did get tested, the results showed that I was HIV positive also. R would come home from work early in the day fatigued. When I tried to discuss it and confront him, he would intimidate me by stating 'he was the doctor, not me.'

"Denial had been a way R dealt with many things in his life, and it would be that way with AIDS. Sometimes I think of him and I'm very angry. If he hadn't denied so much when he began to develop symptoms, he might still be here. But we finally agreed on his getting examined, and he had a lung biopsy as an outpatient. That night we were both at home waiting for a phone call from his doctor. I was in the bathroom and heard the phone ring and knew what it was. I started crying while listening to R on the phone. He was very up, very positive. But when he hung up he, too, started crying. The results were Pneumocystis Carinii Pneumonia (PCP). I went into the next room to be with him. It was a moment so very real. I thought of all the people who had died and what they went through and how this has to be different for us. There will be something to save us. But you can't think of how to handle it. At the same time, however, it was very frightening because we were two people who knew too much.

"We were able to have R treated at home, and not have to enter the hospital. It was always his wish to stay at home, and I was determined to do whatever it took to make him happy. But R was very concerned about people not finding out. Other than his sister and my family, we did not tell any of our friends. I agreed to this but at the same time did not want to handle it this way. After all I've been through, I would not handle it that way today. But at the time, I agreed to play the game.

"R eventually told his employer, and they were very supportive. However, he was very frightened to tell them, afraid to be rejected or thought of as an outcast. In a way, it was almost like coming out to a parent, to tell him or her that he was gay and had AIDS. However, the process was a great relief and a release for him. At that point, he began to deal with AIDS in a healthier way. He was very fortunate to be able to continue doing what he loved — practice medicine. He could sleep at night knowing he had a place to go in the morning, and he felt needed.

"There was a change in his role, and he could not practice medicine 'hands on.' His was one of the first cases his hospital had to deal with, and they were very respectful of him. His position at the hospital changed to that of preceptor, whereby he supervised interns in their patient management. This was a big ego blow to R. He wanted to work to his full potential but he was not okay, and he had to step back, and this was very hard for him to do. He would always have great difficulty in discussing his illness.

"From that point until the summer of 1988, R did fairly well. He continued to work out, we traveled quite a bit, and we managed. We were successful in keeping the diagnosis a secret from our neighbors and most friends. No one ever questioned us or made us feel uncomfortable, even if they did suspect something was wrong. I feel most people have a sense of what is appropriate. We never had to confront that issue, and I'm very thankful for that. For the times R did have to be hospitalized, I treated it as a nonevent and an inconvenience. It was important to deal with him that way. I always had a bag packed, to make it easier when those 'hospital' times came. I tried to have a positive attitude throughout his illness. I did this by treating the disease realistically but did not let it take over our lives.

"Some of the best times we shared together were the simplest of moments. We shared a two-story condo and when R was able to dress himself and walk upstairs to our dining room, we would have dinner together. Now people have dinner together all the time but don't think about how lucky they are. They can eat and drink whatever they want without getting sick or suffering the next few days. Sometime you should share a meal with a loved one and fantasize it's your last. You will realize how much you have to say to one another that has not been expressed before. This experience will change your relationship for the better.

"By Thanksgiving, R's condition had deteriorated. He was incontinent, very weak, having some dementia, and not able to eat very much.

But our neighbors and friends on the block had prepared extravagantly to celebrate the holiday. The food was incredible—wines, liquors, turkey, ham, all kinds of sweets. We would go from apartment to apartment and R needed lots of help going up and down the stairs, and he allowed our friends to assist him. He ate an enormous amount of food, and, although I was concerned, I decided to let him enjoy the evening, and we would deal with what ever happened later.

"When we got home, he was exhausted to the point of not being able to undress. He sat on the bed and wanted to talk. Then he asked me, 'Do you think they know?' It was so hard not to lie, to not want to hurt him, but I had to tell the truth when he asked. After this, he allowed his friends to visit him and to give their support.

"Later that night, he became very sick. It was a combination of the food, his medications, a sudden high temperature and horrible chills. When he finally was in bed and asleep, I knew it would be the last night we would spend in our apartment together. I knew from working with other AIDS patients that he would not get better, and I could not do this anymore by myself. Through this entire journey, I had been self-confident and self-assured, but now I was scared.

"The following day, he was admitted into the hospital and he died a week later. That week, I learned how stress is an enemy in this disease. I had night sweats, my T cells dropped and I had to begin AZT. I knew I was losing R, I was getting sick myself, and I felt there was nowhere to look for hope.

"In the hospital, it was so hard to watch him struggling, in pain, having seizures and being in a coma. All you think about is how to get rid of the pain for him. It finally occurred to me to have him baptized. It took a long time for me to figure it out because I could not hear it, but God was telling me to have him baptized and then he would take him. R died three hours after the priest came.

"I don't believe AIDS is a terminal illness but there comes a time when it turns into one. The last few weeks, the last moments are so difficult. It is a most personal loss to watch someone you love dying every day.

"During the time I cared for R, I was not consciously thinking of my own status of being HIV positive, and so I did a lot of damage to myself. At times, I felt like a string was holding me together. If it wasn't for my family, R's sister and close friends, I could not have managed what I did.

"A most difficult part is when its all over and everyone goes back to their routines. You are in the same environment but you feel purposeless. People are very loving but life goes on, and they forget about you. They want you to feel better, but they don't understand what that entails. Its very hard to begin to take care of yourself; you don't know where your life is. I feel in a way that I'm starting over.

"In the few months after R's death, I made several major life changes. I sold our condo and bought a new home in the south, where I grew up, near my family. I had a roommate for a few months and this was a good transitional step. However, my friends were in the north, and I needed to talk about my experience. AIDS is viewed very differently in the south and not well accepted. At this time, gay life is much more closeted, and people are afraid. I joined a support group and through that began to meet new friends. I became active in the AIDS services organization, and this work is very important to me. Now I am also meeting people outside of these AIDS-centered activities.

"I don't know where I'll end up but I look towards the future, yet at the same time, I take each day as it comes. My goals have changed. This experience helped me to find out what is really important in life, and it's not money, not power, and not position. I've learned to take care of myself, physically, emotionally and spiritually. I live life as though I'll reach 90; you have to have a reason to get up every day. It took awhile to get to this point and it was not easy.

"I am in school now pursuing a degree in counseling. I want to give back what I've been given and to help other people. In a reading assignment for school, I learned about a theory which includes a phase on Generativity. This stage usually occurs in old age, and it is when you give back to society what you have received. I thought, here I am with this disease and I'm in school, not doing what most other people my age are doing. I feel that I've skipped ages 40 to 50, and now I'm 60 and retired.

"Before R died, he talked to me about dating. He wanted me to start to go out before he died, but I did not. But he was giving me permission, and as time goes on, I realize it's okay to feel what I feel about dating. No matter where I go, he will always be with me. Whomever I date will have to understand this. It's not a threat but a part of who I am. I am very proud of that and will never get over him. I am just to a point where I can go out with someone if they understand who I am and what my relationship with R will always mean to me. I want to be free to talk about it in a loving way. Its almost like a test: anyone who can handle that is someone I'll be interested in.

"I feel R and I were put together for a reason. Our relationship together went full circle. He died knowing who he was and who loved him. He learned to let go of unrealistic expectations in life and to forgive the people who had hurt him. He appreciated and understood what love meant and that he didn't have to beg for it. Together we were able to work on issues of denial, and he died a much more self-accepting and fulfilled person.

"When I moved back home to the south, I knew in my heart it was the right thing to do but if it wasn't, I have learned that what is done can be undone. You will find a way to work on how to make it something better.

"My message to you about AIDS is that there are lots of people who care and will support you. It doesn't take the hurt away but they can ease it. If you are going to go on to lead a productive, healthy life you will need the love of your family and friends, so don't shut them out.

"As a way of ending I'd like to share with you a passage from the Book of Genesis, that R often reflected upon, especially in times of stress and difficulty during his life.

> In the beginning God created the heaven and the earth.
>
> And the earth was without form, and void; and darkness was upon the face of the deep. And the Spirit of God moved upon the face of the waters.
>
> And God said, Let there be light: and there was light.
>
> And God saw the light, that it was good: and God divided the light from the darkness.
>
> And God called the light Day, and the Darkness he called Night. And the evening and the morning were the first day. (*The Oxford Self-Pronouncing Bible*, date unknown, p. 7)

DISCUSSION

A gay couple is faced with many complex issues due to AIDS. As highlighted in the case study, the effects of prejudice, fear of disclosure and the need to maintain self-respect have a powerful impact in shaping a couples' response to their crisis. The sense of loss during the disease process can create feelings of helplessness and hopelessness as death becomes imminent. The cycle of secrecy places barriers to support systems but provides a sense of emotional protection. The demands on the caregiver cannot be minimized. Sometimes, in the courageous efforts to support a lover's needs and concerns the caregiver jeopardizes his or her own health physically, mentally, and spiritually. The impact of death, the identity as a single bereaved and moving on are cold realities of life. The process of gay bereavement has unique demands and special issues. Therapists, health care providers and other professionals who are aware of and understand the range of difficulties gay men encounter from homophobia and HIV stigma will be in a position to provide meaningful support and counseling and to assist individuals in their grief work.

CONCLUSION

AIDS has had a devastating effect in the gay community. A majority of the deaths from AIDS in this decade have been gay men. "The increasing number of deaths among gay men caused by AIDS has resulted in an increasing number of survivors who are confronting issues of gay grief" (Klein & Fletcher, 1986). To grieve the loss of a loved one is a profound personal tragedy, and the bereavement process for gay men is intensified due to lack of legal or social status, potential exposure of sexual orientation coupled with the stigma of AIDS, the recent overwhelming number of AIDS-related deaths within the gay community, and concern over their own HIV status. AIDS is a disease that has brought out both the best and the worst in human nature. This paper highlights issues in gay grief, particularly the magnitude of loss experienced.

STUDY QUESTIONS

1. *The face of AIDS is changing from what was once called a Gay disease to that of an international disease that knows no race, color, group or culture. How do you see social acceptance and medical treatment changing in the next decade?*
2. *After a diagnosis of AIDS, suggest an approach that a gay individual might take in sharing his or her homosexuality and HIV status with friends and family.*
3. *What changes, if any, do you see necessary in our social system for surviving spouses of AIDS patients? Analyze this from religious, social, economic, and legal viewpoints.*
4. *Fantasize that today is your last and you have one meal left to share with a significant other. Who would that person be and what subjects, issues, and feelings would you want to talk about and share?*

REFERENCES

Centers for Disease Control, (1989, September). *HIV/AIDS Surveillance*.
Dean, L., Hall, W.E., and Martin, J.L., (1988). Chronic and Intermittent AIDS-Related Bereavement in a Panel of Homosexual Men in New York City. *Journal of Palliative Care 4*, 54-57.

Doka, K.J., (1987). Silent Sorrow: Grief and the Loss of Significant Others. *Death Studies 11*, 455-469.

Greif, G.L., & Porembski, E., (1988). AIDS and Significant Others: Findings from a Preliminary Exploration of Needs. *Health and Social Work 13*, 259-265.

Jones, A., (1988). Nothing Gay About Bereavement. *Nursing Times 84*, 55-57.

Klein, S. & Fletcher, W., (1986). Gay Grief: An Examination of its Uniqueness Brought to Light by the AIDS Crisis. *Journal of Psychosocial Oncology 4*, 15-25.

The Oxford Self-Pronouncing Bible. (Date unknown). New York: The Oxford University Press.

Ruskin, C., (1988). *The Quilt, Stories from The NAMES Project*. (1st ed.). New York: POCKET BOOKS.

Siegal, R.L., & Hoefer, D.D., (1981). Bereavement Counseling for Gay Individuals. *American Journal of Psychotherapy 35*, 51-525.

Tatelbaum, J., (1980). *The Courage to Grieve*. (1st ed.). New York: Lippincott and Crowell.

Resources

Confronting AIDS: Directions for Public Health, Health Care and Research (1986) and *Update: 1988.* National Academy Press, Washington, DC

Understanding AIDS: A Message From the Surgeon General. HHS Publication No. (CDC) HHS-88-8404 (also available in Spanish by calling 1-800-344-SIDA) Available in English by calling 1-800-458-5231

Coping with AIDS. US Department of Health and Human Services. Available free by calling 1-800-458-5231

Report of the Presidential Commission on the Human Immunodeficiency Virus Epidemic. Available for $11.00 from Superintendent of Documents, U.S. Government Printing Office, Washington, DC 20402

Pizzi, M. (Ed.) (March, 1990) American Journal of Occupational Therapy Special Issue on AIDS. Available from the American Occupational Therapy Association, 1383 Piccard Drive, PO Box 1725, Rockville, MD 20850-0822

National AIDS Network. 1012 14th St. N.W. #601, Washington, DC 20005. 202-293-2437

AIDS Hotline, US Public Health Service, Atlanta, GA (24 hours daily) 1-800-342-AIDS

National Gay Task Force (NGTF) 1-800-221-7044 (3-9 p.m.)

National AIDS Information Clearinghouse 1-800-458-5231

Publications Clearinghouse 202-625-8410